Contents

List of contributors

Carol Bates MA, PGCEA, ADM, RM, RN
Education Development Co-ordinator
Education & Research Development
Royal College of Midwives
London

Judy Bothamley MA, PGCEA, ADM, RM, RGN
Senior Lecturer (Midwifery)
Thames Valley University
London

Maureen Boyle MSc, PGCEA, ADM, RM, RGN
Senior Lecturer (Midwifery)
Thames Valley University
London

Joanne Chadwick MSc, PGCEA, ADM, RM, RN
Adjunct Assistant Professor of Maternal and
    Child Health
Boston University
Boston, MA

Helen Crafter MSc, PGCEA, ADM, RM, RGN, FP Cert
Senior Lecturer (Midwifery)
Thames Valley University
London

Debra Kroll MSc, PGCEA, ADM, RM, RN
Lecturer and Practitioner
University College Hospital
London

Michelle Lyne RN, RM, ADM, BEd (Hons)
Lecturer in Midwifery
City University
St Bartholomew School of Nursing and
    Midwifery
London

Sandra McDonald MSc, PGCEA, ADM, RM, RCN
Senior Lecturer (Midwifery)
Thames Valley University
London

Caroline Squire MSc, PGCEA, ADM, RM, RN,
    Lic Ac, Lic OHM
Senior Lecturer (Midwifery)
Thames Valley University
London

Hazel Sundle RM, RGN, Dip HE
Community Midwife
North Tyneside

Margaret Yerby MSc, PGCEA, ADM, RM, RGN
Senior Lecturer (Midwifery)
Thames Valley University
London

Emergencies Around Childbirth

A handbook for midwives

Edited by

Maureen Boyle

Radcliffe Medical Press

Radcliffe Medical Press Ltd
18 Marcham Road
Abingdon
Oxon OX14 1AA
United Kingdom

www.radcliffe-oxford.com
The Radcliffe Medical Press electronic catalogue and online ordering facility.
Direct sales to anywhere in the world.

British Library Cataloguing in Publication Data

A catalogue record for this book is available from the British Library.

ISBN 1 85775 568 5

Typeset by Advance Typesetting Ltd, Oxon
Printed and bound by TJ International Ltd, Padstow, Cornwall

CHAPTER 1

Introduction

Maureen Boyle

As midwives we know that usually pregnancy and birth are normal physiological events. However it is because this is our experience and because most common complications such as postpartum haemorrhages are easily dealt with that many midwives feel less than confident in uncommon or severe life-threatening emergency situations.

This book is intended to provide an easy-to-access resource for practising midwives to enable them to build on their existing understanding of urgent or emergency situations. The importance of extensive knowledge and expertise in high-risk situations goes beyond saving lives in an emergency, important as this is. If adverse events can be predicted and action taken to prevent them, or midwives are ready to deal with them effectively, the likelihood of improving outcomes for mothers and babies is increased. This does not mean that midwives should adopt the medical model of care,[1] but be more concerned with maintaining a wide-ranging and up-to-date knowledge base to ensure normality is maintained as far as possible. If a midwife has considered and reflected on all possible scenarios, including interventions which are appropriate while awaiting assistance, before they arise, she is likely to increase the effectiveness of her actions and her confidence. It is arguable that midwives should practise relevant hands-on skills and the use of study days for this purpose where available is to be encouraged.[2]

It has been identified that a knowledge of critical obstetric problems should be a high priority for obstetricians and that an understanding of the pathophysiology of various conditions and a knowledge of life-saving measures are integral to the effectiveness of treatment.[3] The same must be

the case for midwives, who often have sole responsibility for the care of pregnant women and may be without immediate hospital and medical back-up when an emergency happens.

At first glance, it may be thought that a book about emergencies and high-risk situations around childbirth would give an underlying message that birth is not safe and that the authors would always advocate hospital birth in fully equipped centres. This is not the intended message. On the contrary, it is hoped that by encouraging midwives to enhance their confidence, knowledge and skills to deal with emergencies, a fear of complications would not be a barrier to offering home birth to women. Although the book deals with emergencies which are usually predicted and mean hospitalisation, all events discussed can occur unheralded. It is therefore important that midwives can deal effectively with urgent or emergency situations in the community and for this reason 'first aid' actions are discussed in each chapter.

The need to screen women carefully before advising a home birth has been extensively explored,[4] although the dangers of hospital birth have been less well discussed. Hospital care and the growing number of interventions available may expose healthy women to more risks. In particular emergency caesarean sections may increase the chance of severe obstetric morbidity.[5]

Home births may do much to optimise women's physical and psychological experience of birth, so the slowly increasing trend of home births and the development of birthing centres should be encouraged. A barrier to this trend may be that most recently qualified midwives have never attended a home birth, and this may explain why there is evidence that midwives are not always willing to offer home births to women or do not feel confident in truly autonomous practice.[6,7] For example, many midwives fear maternal collapse whether it is as a result of an easily diagnosed cause such as haemorrhage or of an unknown cause, especially when attending a home birth or in other isolated circumstances.

It is important that midwives feel confident in their knowledge and do not bring anxieties and fears into the birthing environment.[8] Labouring women need to believe in their carers' abilities in order to be relaxed.[9] A good level of knowledge of high- risk conditions is mandatory if midwives are to gain and keep women's confidence. The published letter of a pregnant woman describing how an experienced midwife had asked her 'what is HELLP syndrome?' did nothing to encourage the readers' faith in the midwifery profession.[10]

There is also a case for informed midwifery care, not only in emergency situations, but also when diagnosed obstetric complications have the potential for disaster. Although the obstetrician or other doctor will be the lead professional in such situations, ongoing midwifery care may have beneficial effects on the birth experience, making it seem as normal as possible by providing a focus on pregnancy and impending motherhood rather than on the pathology.

It is most midwives' experience that labour interventions, including unplanned caesarean sections, are becoming more common. It is therefore likely that more women are experiencing physically and/or psychologically traumatic events around the time of birth.

One recent study showed an incidence of 12 cases of severe maternal morbidity for every 1000 deliveries.[5] These potentially life-threatening events may result in long-term physical effects. In more cases women may suffer psychological trauma which can lead to decisions against further pregnancies or the symptoms of post-traumatic stress syndrome. Situations where women experience powerlessness and lack of control are commonly accepted as a forerunner to psychological trauma.[11] Debriefing after the birth is increasingly thought to be important and many midwives feel a postnatal discussion is a vital part of their after-care.[12] Therefore, in many chapters medical interventions not in the midwife's realm have been included, as a review of these procedures may be useful if a midwife needs to discuss these processes with the woman postnatally. No matter how relieved or grateful a woman may feel after

an emergency situation, it would be unlikely that her psychological health would not be improved by being able to make sense of the situation through talking with a knowledgeable midwife.[13]

The *Report on Confidential Enquiries into Maternal Deaths* makes sobering reading and is a useful resource for midwives, especially now they are more fully acknowledged as autonomous care providers.[14] This document is an important source of information and midwives can learn lessons from others' actions in high-risk situations. The latest edition contains a chapter on midwifery practice and, amongst other issues, discusses midwifery accountability and advocacy, stating that they have a responsibility to challenge medical decisions when they believe that to be in the interests of the women in their care. All midwives would consider this to be good practice. This book contains much information that will enable midwives to update their knowledge on high-risk medical/obstetrical situations which occur only infrequently. Although maternal mortality in the UK is now statistically low, the number of deaths where sub-standard care is implicated is too high for any complacency in those who care for women during childbirth.

The *Seventh Annual Confidential Enquiry into Stillbirths and Deaths in Infancy*[15] identified a need for knowledgeable practitioners to deal with breech delivery at home, the majority of which will be unexpected. Since most breech presentations are now born by caesarean section midwives rarely experience vaginal breech births. There is therefore a clear need for midwives to regularly review this subject to ensure their skills are up-to-date, especially if they lack practical experience.

The *Eighth Confidential Enquiry into Stillbirths and Deaths in Infancy*[16] identified not only failures to act appropriately in high-risk situations, but also a lack of recognition of some high-risk situations. Again, frequent review of uncommon events will make them more readily identifiable to midwives. For this reason the book contains a chapter on the less usual conditions that could complicate pregnancies as well as chapters on the most common emergencies or high-risk situations.

A chapter on risk assessment is also included given that appropriate risk assessment and considered midwifery interventions may reduce the number of emergency situations. It also contains relevant information on litigation, because this is an area of concern to many midwives, especially following emergency situations.

This book has been written by midwives for midwives, however the content is unsurprisingly very medically weighted. Nevertheless, it is hoped by all the authors that this information will be used by midwives, not only to perhaps save lives and prevent morbidity, but also to enable women's experiences to become more fulfilling overall, as they are cared for by confident and knowledgeable midwives.

References

1 Bryar R (1995) *Theory for Midwifery Practice.* MacMillan, Basingstoke.

2 Jevor P and Stewart S (2001) Delivery suite emergencies. *Pract Midwife.* **4** (8): 14–16.

3 Van Geign H and Vothknecht S (1996) Training in the management of critical problems: teacher's view. *Eur J Obstet Gynaecol Repro Biol.* **65** (1): 145–8.

4 Campbell R (1999) Review and assessment of selection criteria used when booking pregnant women at different places of birth. *Br J Obstet Gynaecol.* **106** (6): 550–6.

5 Waterstone M, Bewley S and Wolfe C (2001) Incidence and predictors of severe obstetric morbidity: case-control study. *BMJ.* **322**: 1089–94.

6 Magill-Cuerden J (2001) A holiday in Devon: the RCM congress. *Br J Midwif.* **9** (6): 346–7.

7 Floyd L (1995) Community midwives' views and experience of home birth. *Midwif.* **11**: 3–10.

8 Weston R (2001) When birth goes wrong. *Pract Midwife.* **4** (8): 10–12.

9 Green J, Curtis P, Price H and Renfrew M (1998) *Continuing to Care.* Books for Midwives Press, Cheshire.

10 Thompson T (1997) I knew more about HELLP than specialist midwife. *Action on Pre-eclampsia (APEC) Newsletter* **14**: 7–8.

11 Green J, Coupland V and Kitzinger J (1998) *Great Expectations: a prospective study of women's expectations and experiences of childbirth* (2e). Books for Midwives Press, Cheshire.

12 Hammett P (1997) Midwives and debriefing. In: M Kirkham and E Perkins (eds) *Reflections on Midwifery.* Bailliere Tindall, London.

13 Axe S (2000) Labour debriefing is crucial for good psychological care. *Br J Midwif.* **8** (10): 626–31.

14 Lewis G (ed) (2001) *Why Mothers Die 1997–1999: the 5th report of the confidential enquiries into maternal deaths in the United Kingdom.* RCOG Press, London.

15 Maternal and Childbirth Research Consortium (2000) *Confidential Enquiry into Stillbirth and Deaths in Infancy* (Seventh Annual Report). CESDI, London.

16 Maternal and Childbirth Research Consortium (2001) *Confidential Enquiry into Stillbirth and Deaths in Infancy* (Eighth Annual Report). CESDI, London.

CHAPTER 2

Maternal and neonatal resuscitation

Margaret Yerby

Maternal resuscitation

The necessity to resuscitate a pregnant woman or new mother is not an expected event. The *Advisory Statement* produced by the International Liaison Committee on Resuscitation[1] quotes the occurrence of cardiac arrest in pregnancy as 1:30 000 deliveries.

Can cardiac arrest in pregnancy be predicted? Recognising certain complications of pregnancy that place women at risk can help clinicians in predicting collapse in some circumstances. Some of these complications are (*see also* Chapter 11):

- amniotic fluid embolism

- pulmonary embolism

- eclampsia

- drug toxicity (magnesium sulphate, bupivacaine)

- congestive cardiomyopathy

- aortic dissection

- trauma and haemorrhage (leading to hypovolaemia).

The most common causes of cardiopulmonary arrest are eclampsia (*see* Chapter 4) and hypovolaemia.[2] Hypovolaemia is caused through excessive blood loss at delivery or indeed at any time in pregnancy or afterwards, creating an imbalance in the circulatory system.

If the mother collapses and is in a shocked state evaluation of all the body systems has to be made in order to decide the way forward, as resuscitative measures may have to be taken. Box 2.1 lists the principles of care when this emergency takes place.

Box 2.1: Principles of care following collapse

- Early identification of the problems.

- Maintenance of oxygen levels.

- Maintenance of fluid levels.

- Maintenance of circulation.

- Prevention of multiple organ failure.

- Evaluation of fetal condition.

As pregnancy is very much a family event it must not be forgotten that relatives may be close at hand and the partner, in particular, may well be present at maternal collapse. The effects upon the psychological well-being of these onlookers must also be considered. Admission to the intensive care unit is a matter of course once cardiopulmonary arrest has occurred in order that intensive therapy may be carried out. Close relatives need sensitive support at this time from both midwives and doctors.

Physiological events leading up to and following arrest

Collapse of the woman may present initially as a condition of shock. She may exhibit a rapid but thready pulse, low blood pressure and pale sweaty skin. Consciousness may be impaired or she may seem disorientated. Total collapse may then occur. The heart will stop beating, respiration will cease and unless resuscitation takes place within three minutes irreversible damage will take place. For survival, the pumping action of the heart needs to be sustained to maintain blood circulation around the body to oxygenate the tissues in the body. It is imperative to maintain the woman's vital body systems.

Effective treatment of the woman will also treat the foetus. If treatment of the woman is impossible, it has been documented that delivery must occur within four minutes of the mother's death to save the foetus.[2,3]

Delivery of the baby may benefit the mother as this will improve maternal cardiac output, and stroke volume by some 30% and enable better recovery.[4] Resuscitation is more effective without the foetus *in utero*.

Adaptive changes in physiology in pregnancy

The adaptation of maternal systems in pregnancy will alter the response of the mother to collapse. For example, in severe blood loss the maternal blood pressure and pulse respond more slowly to a circulatory insult. By the time the maternal systems show the traditional responses to hypovolaemia (tachycardia and low blood pressure) the woman will be in a severe crisis and may need more intensive therapy to survive.

Cardiac output increases in the first four weeks of pregnancy, which in turn increases the pulse rate. This is in response to an increase in blood volume, which is caused mainly by an increase in plasma volume. The blood supply to the uterus increases from 60 ml per minute to approximately 600 ml per minute at term. The increase in blood volume affects atrial naturetic peptide (ANP) because the heart senses the greater volume with stretch receptors which increase ANP. ANP encourages more excretion of fluid from the kidneys and acts as a diuretic.[5] These physiological changes may mask the effect of shock in the pregnant woman. Therefore it is important to replace fluid early on and to be prepared for collapse, rather than to wait for the normal signs and symptoms of hypovolaemia in the pregnant trauma patient.

Physiological changes when body systems are not sustained

When the heart stops beating circulation of blood stops, all the cells in the body become hypoxic and cell metabolism alters to create an acidosis. Blood pH should be maintained at between 7.0 and 7.4. At cellular level, metabolism requires oxygen to produce adenosine triphosphate (ATP), the energy source to power the cells' functions, the end products being carbon dioxide and water. Carbon dioxide is normally a respiratory stimulant but a build-up of it in a situation where a woman has collapsed is detrimental to the balance of body fluids. Without constant delivery of fluid via the circulatory system cellular function becomes anaerobic and causes acidosis. The respiratory system fails, the blood does not get supplied with oxygen, and carbon dioxide builds up in the capillary beds and is not excreted. The kidneys are no longer supplied with filtrate or oxygen to assist them to break down excess substrates in the blood, maintain a balance and excrete harmful substances. The brain is unable to function without oxygen and cell death quickly occurs. The arterial base deficit measurement of blood depicts the available buffering solutions in the blood that could correct the acid base balance physiologically (the normal range being between –2 to +2 mmol/l). Lactate levels measure acidosis and normally are <2.5 mmol/l of blood. These measurements are easily tested in the laboratory, but lactate levels may alter in relation to liver damage or sepsis, as clearance is not so efficient.[6] Normal blood values are given in Box 2.2. It is important to

---

Box 2.2: Normal blood levels

- Lactate <2.5 mmol/l.
- Base deficit –2 to +2 mmol/l.
- pH 7.2.
- pCO_2 50 mmHg.
- pO_2 40 mmHg.

consider that blood circulation and respiration must be maintained with an adequate circulating fluid volume for the body to survive cardio-pulmonary collapse.[7]

In pregnancy postural hypotension is created when the woman is in the dorsal position for periods of time. It occurs from the second trimester onwards and as the foetus grows it becomes more of a problem. During pregnancy large amounts of blood pool in the peripheral circulation. If the woman is in labour and has an epidural analgesic for pain relief the situation will be exacerbated because the sympathetic nervous system has been paralysed to facilitate pain relief and thus venous return is impaired. Traditionally resuscitation would be performed on a patient in the dorsal position. In the pregnant woman it is important to maintain venous return and good circulation, so the wedge position, which is a left lateral tilt, is used (*see* Figures 2.1 and 2.2). Following trauma it is important to consider the possibility of neck injury and to immobilise the neck prior to tilting the pregnant patient.[8]

Principles of life support in pregnancy

Because the need for cardiopulmonary resuscitation is rare in pregnancy little has been specifically written on the support of women who collapse and require it. Guidelines must be taken from the principles of adult life support laid down by the American Heart Association[9] and the Resuscitation Council (UK).[10] Midwives should keep up to date with the requirements for cardiopulmonary resuscitation (CPR) by attending yearly sessions organised in most units by the anaesthetic depart-ment. A multidisciplinary approach to care in this area is paramount and communication is the key to efficient organisation. The maternity department should be fully equipped despite the rare occur-rence of CPR. The equipment should be regularly checked to ensure it is ready to facilitate resus-citation if and when the need arises. *See* Boxes 2.3 and 2.4 for detail on resuscitation equipment. In any life-threatening event it is important to remember that help is required. This can usually be obtained by ringing for an ambulance and para-medic assistance if the woman is outside the hos-pital or by activating the emergency bell in a hospital situation to summon other midwives who will then request the cardiac arrest team. If the cardiac arrest occurs outside the hospital it is important to phone for help first, before commencing resus-citation. It is imperative to obtain medical aid as soon as possible because outcomes are better if defibrillation occurs earlier rather than later.[11]

At the first signs of collapse a pregnant woman should be immediately turned to the left lateral

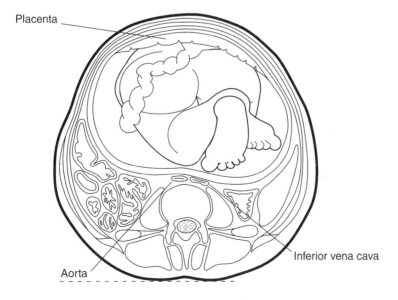

Figure 2.1 Aortal and inferior vena caval compression in dorsal position

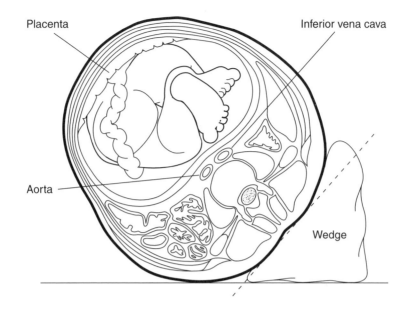

Figure 2.2 Left lateral tilt relieves compression

Box 2.3: Resuscitation equipment available in hospital

Equipment ready for use on top of trolley

- Portable oxygen and relevant masks.
- Laerdal masks.
- Mask and rebreathing bag attached to oxygen.
- Electrocardiograph (ECG) pads to attach to patient.
- Suction catheter.
- Defibrillation pads.

Other equipment (in drawers)

- Endotracheal tubes (ET) in various sizes.
- Gel.
- Airways.
- Intróducer for *ET* tubes.
- Scissors.

Intravenous equipment

- Cannulae.
- Giving sets.

Intravenous fluids

- Dextrose 5%.
- Sodium chloride 0.9%.
- Gelufusin.
- Cut down set.
- Small ampoules of sodium chloride.

Drugs (in sealed, dated boxes)

- Atropine.
- Adrenaline.
- Adenosine.
- Calcium chloride 10%.
- Diazemols.
- Glucose 5%.
- Lidocaine 2%.
- Narcan®.
- Sodium bicarbonate 8.4%.
- Verapamil.

Box 2.4: Resuscitation equipment available at home births

- Portable oxygen.

- Laerdal mask.

- Ambubags.

- Portable suction.

- Cannulae and giving sets.

- Intravenous fluids.

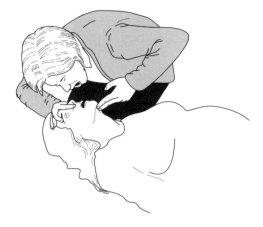

Figure 2.3 Head position for mouth-to-mouth ventilation

position and firmly wedged at a left tilt using pillows or a foam wedge. This will aid venous return and prevent postural hypotension. If pillows or foam are not available an assistant can kneel behind the woman to act as a wedge and stabilise the left tilt position. The basic principles of ABC prevail:

- A – airway

- B – breathing

- C – circulation.

The airway can be maintained by:

- tilting the head by applying pressure on the forehead with one hand and pushing the chin up with the finger tips of the other hand

- then pinching the nose with the thumb and forefinger of the hand that was on the forehead to prevent air escaping when artificial respiration is performed (*see* Figure 2.3)

- performing a jaw thrust manoeuvre if the airway is still obstructed by finding the angle of the jaw with the fingers and pushing in an upward and forward movement.

Oxygenation should be established in the first instance with mouth-to-mouth resuscitation, using a laerdal mask if available, by giving two good breaths into the lungs. It should be continued until further medical aid is available. Once an airway is established and a recovery made it is essential to observe the woman's condition and administer oxygen with a mask that fits well (*see* Figure 2.4). If the patient has sustained any trauma to the neck, care should be taken not to

over extend the neck until an x-ray has ruled out any neck problems.

To continue the resuscitation process after skilled help arrives, the airway needs to be maintained and an endotracheal tube inserted. This could be difficult as changes in pregnancy can cause oedema of the neck tissues or the glottis and therefore enlargement of the neck. To prevent problems an experienced obstetric anaesthetist should insert the tube. Cricoid pressure during intubation will prevent the acid contents of the stomach, which may not be empty, from blocking the airway.

Cardiac compression should be undertaken, with the pregnant woman in the left tilt position, and in the knowledge that the heart is displaced to the left in pregnancy. If available, two people should give initial life support until the arrest team arrives. To perform cardiac compression, locate the lower ribs with the fingers of one hand and then slide the fingers up the edge of the ribs to the sternum. With the other hand, trace down the sternum and place the heel of that hand next to the fingers locating the sternum. Lock the hands together, straighten the arms and, placing weight on the hands from vertically above the woman, press down for 15 compressions (*see* Figure 2.5). Repeat this action about 100 times a minute depressing the sternum 4–5 cm each time. The ratio with two people would be 15:2 (compressions to breaths), continuing until the multidisciplinary team arrive with the equipment.[12]

If alone it may be necessary to commence resuscitation with the ratio of one breath to five

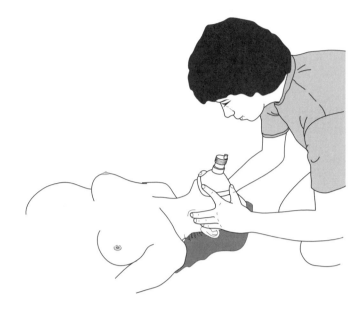

Figure 2.4 Head position for performing mouth-to-mask ventilation

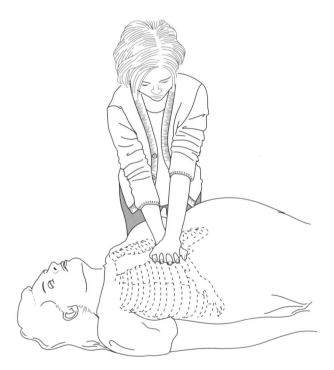

Figure 2.5 Hand position for chest compression

chest compressions. It is important to get medical aid before starting resuscitation as defibrillation may be required. Once started the lone rescuer may feel unable to give up rescue attempts to call for help even though support is needed from others in order to be successful. It is always better to work as a team of two people so that the lungs are inflated more effectively.[12] For a quick recap of basic life support action *see* Box 2.5.

Throughout the rescue attempt observations for signs of life should be made as recently discussed at the Guidelines 2000 Conference.[13] The signs to look for are movement or spontaneous breathing. At the onset of arrest the condition of the mother is paramount and the chances of saving the woman and the foetus depend on successful maternal life support. Therefore the condition of the mother will take precedence over the foetal condition.[8]

Defibrillation

Once resuscitation has commenced the heart may be working erratically and defibrillation to stabilise heart action will be required. If the ventricular pumping action is not stabilised within two minutes, rescue attempts will not be successful as the pumping action of the heart is necessary not only for general circulation but also to supply oxygen to the myocardium of the heart.[15] Paddles are placed on the sternum and to the left of the chest wall (midaxillary between the fifth and sixth ribs) and an electric shock is then passed

Box 2.5: Basic adult life support actions

- Check conscious state (shake and shout).

- Clear airway (head tilt, chin lift).

- Check breathing (look and listen).

- Two effective breaths (watch chest for movement).

- Check circulation (10 sec) or spontaneous movement.

- No circulation: chest compressions at 100 per minute.

- Ratio with two people: 15 compressions to 2 breaths.

- Ratio with one person: 10 compressions to 2 breaths.

Adapted from *Advanced Life Support Manual.*[12]

through the heart (*see* Figure 2.6). It is important to ensure all personnel have no contact with the woman while she is being shocked. Currents of 300 J have been shown to be safe to use in pregnancy.[14,16]

It is envisaged that automated defibrillators will become accessible to all first aiders in all work places to improve outcomes of arrests outside hospitals. These defibrillators analyse the rhythm of the heart and give an automatically measured current to the patient. They are easy to use and are 100% fail-safe.[12]

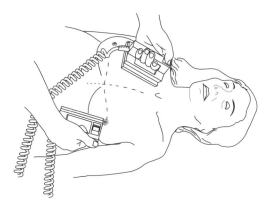

Figure 2.6 Chest and paddle positions for defibrillation

Fluid replacement

At the first signs of a woman's condition deteriorating measures should be taken to prevent it worsening by administering intravenous fluids. In a community setting the midwife could commence giving fluids intravenously if she has the equipment, but if not the paramedic will do so on arrival. Once an arrest has taken place defibrillation and drugs (*see* Box 2.6) should be given alternately, whilst support of respiration and cardiac output is continued. An essential component of this support is the use of intravenous fluids, as inadequate perfusion creates a metabolic acidosis and if the base deficit and lactate are not stabilised adult respiratory distress syndrome (ARDS) may result. As a guide, women with a base deficit of <6 mmol/l are more likely to suffer ARDS and its consequent multiple organ failure.

The aim of fluid replacement is to balance the chemical components of the blood and to maintain blood pressure if it is low. However in

---

Box 2.6: Drugs used to support systems following the arrival of the multidisciplinary team

Adrenaline (epinephrine)

- Given intravenously or into the tracheal tube.

- Adrenaline is a sympathomimetic drug which increases the heart rate and its force of contraction which improves blood flow to the vital organs.

- It is the first medication to be administered in an arrest situation. However its use in pregnancy does mean that blood is drawn away from the uterus thus affecting utero-placental perfusion.[14]

Atropine

- Given intravenously.

- Atropine blocks the action of the vagus nerve on the sinoatrial node and atrioventricular node thus improving heart conduction in hypotension and bradycardia.[12]

Lignocaine (lidocaine)

- Given intravenously: bolus followed by infusion.

- Lignocaine stabilises ventricular fibrillation and prevents ectopic activity or extra beats in the ventricles.

- It is not effective in the management of atrial arrhythmias.

- Overdose of lignocaine causes drowsiness, confusion and muscular twitching which can be quickly reversed by discontinuing the drug.[12]

Amiodarone

- This drug has been shown in a clinical trial to be effective in arrests outside hospital and also in situations when ventricular fibrillation had not been successfully treated with defibrillation. However it was not compared with lidocaine as its actions are similar.[12]

---

itself this can be detrimental as it could alter the body's thermal balance and disturb blood clots. Crystalloids such as normal saline, 5% dextrose and dextrose saline have been shown to reduce blood viscosity, lower haematocrit and dilute clotting factors, so it is important to control haemorrhage prior to infusion with fluids.[17] The quicker normal blood patterns are stabilised, the better the outcome. It is important to maintain careful records of fluids used in an emergency situation and be aware of the dangers of overloading the woman's system.

Support and outcomes

The first part of this chapter deals with cardiac resuscitation of the pregnant woman, but little has been said regarding possible outcomes for the mother or the family. At best, resuscitation will be successful with full recovery of the mother and the birth of a healthy baby. At worst, the family may experience not only the loss of a loved one, but also the loss of the unborn baby. They may have observed the collapse and death, and the effect this may have on their grief process may be profound.

This subject is not easily researched or indeed written about. However when questioned some relatives have said that they preferred to stay while resuscitation attempts were made, regardless of the consequences of the procedure. It helped them to come to terms with the death of the loved one if that was the outcome. Support is all-important here and it is imperative that a member of staff is available to discuss and explain events, if possible while they are happening.[13,18,19]

A relevant report by a sister who witnessed her brother's accident and subsequent attempted resuscitation was published in the *British*

Medical Journal.[20] She was very positive about the fact that she had been with her brother and stated that she had discussed the processes involved with doctors and nurses who were divided in their opinions as to the advantages and disadvantages of the observation of resuscitation procedures by relatives. Such involvement may help the grief process, but it may be difficult for health professionals to see the benefits at the time. Perhaps professionals need to openly discuss this subject and review policy on the involvement of relatives at resuscitation events.

Midwives should also give support to each other as the necessity for resuscitation of a mother is such a rare and tragic occurrence that it is very distressing for all concerned.

Neonatal resuscitation

The birth of a baby always brings anticipation and a sense of achievement on completion, and it is expected that the baby will cry or gasp. This is the natural reflex for a baby entering the world as its chest walls, having been squeezed by the vagina, are suddenly released and lung expansion can take place. As the baby begins to breathe, oxygen permeates the cells and the skin colour changes from blue to pink in minutes.

On occasions and sometimes totally unexpectedly there is silence in the room as the baby is born. A baby with cyanosed skin may give a quiet gasp. If a good heartbeat can be felt or heard, circulation has been maintained but there may still be no good cry or signs of respiration. This is a scenario every midwife will recognise and fear.

The list of conditions which increase risk for the neonate is formidable (*see* Box 2.7) but gives the practitioner some guidance on when resuscitation of a neonate or transfer of a mother in labour to hospital may become necessary. All events, including conditions which increase risk, are required to be recorded in the mother's notes and it has been reported in many situations where a baby has died that such communication is of importance in the prevention of neonatal death.[22]

Midwives therefore need to keep up to date with neonatal resuscitation skills. This is particularly important because 70% of all normal births are supervised by midwives and so they are often the first professional to diagnose collapse in the

---

Box 2.7: Conditions which increase risk for the neonate

Antepartum factors

- Maternal history of medical disease, e.g. diabetes, hypertension, heart disease.
- Pre-eclampsia.
- Anaemia or isoimmunisation.
- Previous foetal or neonatal death.
- Haemorrhage in the second or third trimesters.
- Maternal infection.
- Increase or decrease in liquor volume.
- Pre- or post-term gestation.
- Multiple pregnancy.
- Maternal substance abuse, e.g. drugs, alcohol or smoking.
- Foetal abnormality.
- No antenatal care.
- Age <16 or >35.

Intrapartum factors

- Abruptio placentae or placenta praevia.
- Prolapsed cord.
- Pre-term labour.
- Precipitous labour.
- Prolonged labour >24 hours.
- Prolonged rupture of membranes >18 hours.
- Prolonged second stage of labour >2 hours.
- Abnormal presentation or malposition of the foetus.
- Forceps or ventouse extraction.
- Emergency caesarean section or general anaesthesia.
- Abnormal uterine action, leading to uterine atony.
- Meconium-stained liquor.
- Narcotics administered to the mother within 4 hours of birth.
- Abnormal heart rate patterns on cardiotocography (CTG).

Adapted from the ILCOR[21]

newborn and instigate resuscitation.[23] The *Confidential Enquiry into Stillbirths and Deaths in Infancy*[22] stated that in '95% of responding units all midwives regularly attend neonatal resuscitation skills sessions'.

Intrapartum and the foetus

In utero the foetus is protected by membranes and liquor; the placenta is its life support system. The foetus obtains oxygen from maternal oxygen supplies via the placenta and if these are inadequate at any time the heart rate patterns of the foetus change. The lungs, heart and some components of the blood of the foetus are adapted to survive in this enclosed environment (*see* Box 2.8).

There are three principle shunts (*see* Box 2.8) which facilitate a good supply of oxygen to the vital organs. When the blood enters the system from the placenta oxygenation is high, but it soon mixes with the blood already in circulation which has less oxygen. The shunts within the system ensure that the vital organs obtain higher levels of oxygen saturated blood from the heart as quickly as possible.[24] As the foetus receives oxygen from the mother it also transfers excreted products to her. This momentarily alters pH values in the mother and permits greater levels of oxygen to

---

Box 2.8: Foetal adaptation *in utero*

Heart

- Ventricles pump in parallel.

Three principle shunts

- Ductus venosus: diverts highly-oxygenated blood to the inferior vena cava.

- Foramen ovale: diverts highly-oxygenated blood to the left side of the heart in order to supply the body.

- Ductus arteriosus: diverts blood away from the non-expanding lungs to the aorta.

Blood

- Higher haemoglobin levels which have a higher binding capacity to oxygen because of its structure (foetal haemoglobin).

---

diffuse across to the foetus (the Bohr effect).[7] In addition haemoglobin content is higher in foetal blood, which therefore attracts more oxygen.

As labour commences the delivery of oxygen to the foetus may be affected. Uterine contractions may affect the volume of blood circulating at placental level and/or the cord may become trapped between the pelvis and soft tissues during the descent of the foetus. The healthy foetus will automatically react to this disruption by an alteration in heart rate which is brought about by the baroreceptors in the aortic arch and carotid sinuses which sense the partial pressure of oxygen dissolved in blood plasma. The chemoreceptors in the peripheral and brain systems are sensitive to blood pH levels.[7] A variable heart rate therefore indicates the foetus' ability to adapt to varying circumstances. A transitory rise in heart rate may indicate intrauterine asphyxia and would mean a degree of stress for the foetus. It is expected that the preterm foetus has a higher heart rate which becomes more stable with maturity.

The level of acidosis is important when assessing foetal well-being in labour. Levels over 7.25 are normal, those between 7.20 and 7.25 are viewed as pre-acidotic and levels below 7.20 indicate acidosis. The level of acidosis indicates the level of lactic acid in the foetal systems which rises due to lack of oxygen and an increase in carbon dioxide levels in the bloodstream. This indicates hypoxia *in utero*.[25]

The slow rise to the baseline rate following a bradycardial incident indicates the return of more adequate oxygen levels for the foetus.[26] The mature foetus that is stressed will often pass meconium and this is brought about by the over production of motilin, a bowel hormone which increases gut motility in these circumstances.[27]

All observations of the foetal condition by whatever means are important. Abnormal findings will alert the midwife to the fact that the foetus may require earlier rather than later delivery. However there are some situations (*see* Box 2.9) in which the midwife will need to observe the foetus even more carefully in labour in anticipation of problems at birth. Foetal distress and/or meconium stained liquor are warning signs in labour that would influence the midwife's decision to transfer the mother to hospital and to call for a paediatrician when birth is imminent.

At birth the transition to extrauterine life occurs almost instantly. The occlusion of the cord alters pressures in the right side of the heart and the infant's first breath fills the lungs with air.[5] If the baby does not take that first breath (*see* Box 2.9 for reasons for failure to do so) the midwife should instigate closer observation and ensure resuscitative measures are commenced promptly.

Box 2.9: Reasons for failure of the newborn to commence respiration

- Adverse intrapartum events, e.g. difficult labour, foetal distress.
- Drugs given to the mother.
- Immaturity.
- Sepsis.
- Abnormalities of the respiratory system, i.e. diaphragmatic hernia, obstruction.
- Trauma.

Adapted from Drew et al.[28]

The Apgar score (*see* Table 2.1) is the traditional assessment of newborn well-being. A scoring

system based on points out of ten assesses heart rate, respiratory effort, muscle tone, reflex response and colour. It is a quick and easy assessment of the newborn's condition at birth made at one and five minutes (and at ten minutes if necessary) and provides a guide to further development in the neonate's systems. The reliability of the Apgar score versus readings of the pH of the umbilical arterial blood at birth in respect of success in predicting adverse neonatal outcomes has been questioned, but has been proved to be an appropriate assessment tool.[29]

The room must be prepared prior to birth. A warm atmosphere is very important. All relevant equipment should be checked and maintained, especially when a birth is expected. As the baby is born, the midwife should dry it and observe its overall condition. In many circumstances the baby may be delivered into the mother's arms and then dried. If the baby does not show signs of respiratory effort and continues to remain cyanosed the ABC of resuscitation should be followed.[30] Box 2.10 lists the immediate measures to take when a baby does not spontaneously commence respiration, and are the basic requirements to stabilise its condition.[21]

Table 2.1: Apgar scoring system[28]

Sign	Score 0	1	2
Heart rate	Absent	<100 beats/minute	>100 beats/minute
Respiratory effort	Absent	Weak, irregular	Strong, regular
Reflex response	None	Weak movement	Cry
Colour	Blue or pale	Body pink, extremities blue	Completely pink
Muscle tone	Limp	Partial flexion	Active movement

Box 2.10: Action plan for active resuscitation[8,21]

- Dry the baby observing the Apgar score at this time.
- Clear the airway, opening it with a head tilt. It is important not to over stimulate by deep suction at the oral pharyngeal level as this may prevent spontaneous respiratory effort.
- Administer oxygen by mask.
- Observe the apex beat: if >100 beats per minute, observe for spontaneous recovery; if <60 beats per minute, cardiac massage should be commenced.
- If there is no spontaneous recovery, help is urgently required.
- Advanced life support will be necessary.

The Paediatric Working Group suggest that 'approximately 5–10% of the newborn require some degree of active resuscitation at birth'.[21] For example, in a labour ward delivering twenty babies a day this would mean that two of those babies would require active resuscitation – a sobering thought and one that emphasises the necessity for every midwife to be competent in resuscitation skills.

Advanced life support in the newborn

Warmth

It is necessary to maintain the baby's temperature at a constant level, as a drop in temperature will mean that stored glucose will be used to produce more heat to raise the temperature and the neonate will require more oxygen to efficiently carry out cell metabolism.[7]

Ventilation

A face mask with a pressure bag is the most common form of early ventilation once the airway is cleared (see Figure 2.7).[28] In the presence of meconium, it has been traditional to suction a baby under direct vision after endotracheal intubation to clear thick meconium from the vocal chords and prevent meconium aspiration syndrome. However a recent Cochrane review has suggested that it is not necessary to intubate and suction the 'vigorous term infant' as there seem to be no benefits to outcomes over

and above oropharyngeal suction. The studies included four randomised controlled trials and suggested that more research was needed in this area to give clinicians more definitive data.[31]

Position the baby's head to achieve the optimum airway opening (see Figure 2.8). Masks used for ventilation should fit the baby well by not occluding the eyes or overlapping the chin. If the mask does not fit correctly oxygen pressure will not be maintained and delivery will be poor. An unimpeded airway should be maintained by lifting the chin whilst maintaining a good fit with the mask. Chest movement should be observed and when respiration is adequate, the colour and heart rate of the baby should be assessed. When the heart rate is more than 100 beats per minute, ventilation can be stopped and the baby returned to the mother. If the baby continues to be slow to respire independently, the administration of naloxone should be considered if narcotics were given in the last four hours before delivery. It is also worth checking again that the airway is clear.

Endotracheal intubation should be carried out if initial bag-and-mask ventilation has failed or if meconium aspiration is thought to have occurred in a baby that is not responding. A preterm baby may be difficult to resuscitate because an inadequate quantity of surfactant lining makes the lungs 'stiff'. By this time if a midwife is still without medical assistance, it should be sought as a matter of urgency. Intubation is not difficult but requires to be undertaken by someone proficient in its use.[21] The principles of intubation are given in Box 2.11.

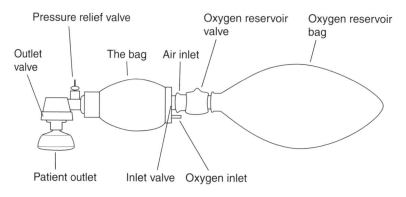

Pressure relief valve   Oxygen reservoir valve   Oxygen reservoir bag

Outlet valve   The bag   Air inlet

Patient outlet   Inlet valve   Oxygen inlet

Figure 2.7 Mask

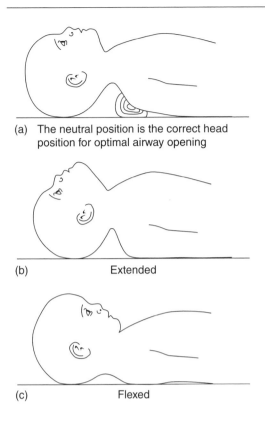

(a) The neutral position is the correct head position for optimal airway opening

(b) Extended

(c) Flexed

Figure 2.8 Head position for optimum airway opening

Cardiac compression

Throughout the ventilation procedure observation of the heart rate should continue. If the rate is less than 60 beats per minute, chest compressions should commence. *See* Figure 2.9 for the recommended finger positions. Neonatal asphyxia causes an imbalance in tissue oxygenation causing an acidosis. Ventilating the baby with adequate oxygen may enable it to establish respiration. If the heart is not adequately perfusing the tissues, chest compression will increase the heart rate so that oxygen permeates the cells throughout the body and stabilises metabolism. Chest compressions should not be commenced before ventilation.[21] *See* Box 2.12 for the basic principles.

Following the commencement of chest compression and ventilation, assessment of vital signs should be made at 30-second intervals. If the heart rate continues to be below 60 beats per minute, the administration of drugs to stimulate the baby would be the next step. The insertion of a direct line via the umbilical vein or administration via an endotracheal tube are the best routes.

The equipment usually available in a hospital for neonatal resuscitation is listed in Box 2.13.

Home birth

In the home situation it would be unusual to encounter problems in the newborn baby following a normal birth. Drugs are always minimally used and labour is usually normal and straightforward. It is a good principle to bear in mind that one midwife should be responsible for the care of the baby at a home birth.

Box 2.11: Principles of intubation[28]

- The equipment includes a straight-bladed laryngoscope with a size 1 blade.

- Check the bulb before use.

- Lay the baby on a flat surface with the neck in a neutral position.

- Hold the laryngoscope in the left hand and hold the head steady with the right.

- Insert the blade until the glottis can be seen; over-ride the glottis.

- Lift the blade upwards and forwards (the vocal chords should be in view).

- Now insert the tracheal tube, but only if the chords are relaxed; if the chords are in spasm and closed, do not force the tube down.

- Once the tube is inserted, ventilate and check that the lungs are inflating and the baby's colour is improving.

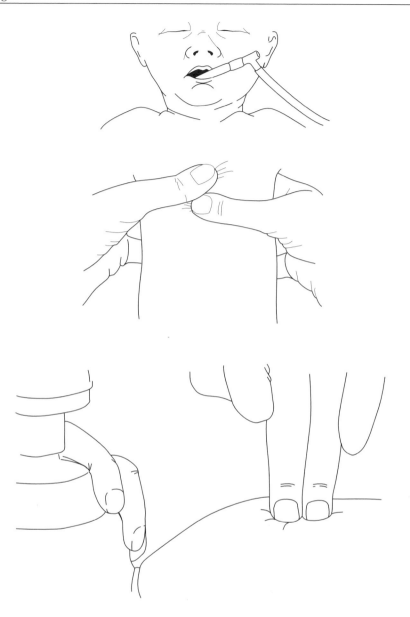

Figure 2.9 Finger positions for chest compression

If necessary the midwife would immediately dry the baby, which would give stimulation, wrap it in warm towels and administer oxygen, observing the heart rate and respiratory effort. A clear airway is essential, but it is important that suction is gentle. If immediate recovery does not take place, the call for emergency backup is vital. While this is coming, respiration should be assisted with a mask and bag. These initial ventilations are important if the baby has shown little respiratory effort as the lungs need to inflate for the anatomical changes in the lungs and heart to be completed. If the heart is beating at less than 60 beats per minute, chest compressions should be commenced on a 3:1 ratio.

Resuscitation at home is fraught with problems, including the lack of equipment (*see* Box 2.14 for essentials), isolation from advanced medical

Box 2.12: Principles of chest compression and ventilation[21]

- Ratio of chest compression to ventilation: 3:1.

- Place two thumbs on the lower third of the sternum, hands encircling the chest (the preferred position) or place two fingers on the sternum at right angles to the chest.

- The depth of compression should be one third of the chest anterior-posterior diameter.

- Compression must be strong enough to feel a palpable pulse.

- Aim to deliver 90 compressions to 30 breaths/min.

- Assess the condition at 30 second intervals and continue until the pulse (usually femoral) rate >60 beats/min.

Box 2.13: Resuscitation equipment available in hospital[28]

- A resuscitaire with a flat bed, an overhead heater and light. A Tom Thumbs, apparatus fixed to the wall and available in the room: may be preferable to a resuscitaire as it is less cumbersome and may be less frightening for the family.

- Fluid chart.

- Drug chart.

- Infant's notes.

To maintain the airway

- Suction, not exceeding minus 100 mmHg.

- Suction catheters in sizes 6, 8 and 10 FG.

- Oropharyngeal airways in sizes 0 and 00.

- Nasogastric tubes.

For ventilation

- Self inflating bag and mask (Laerdal bag).

- Face masks in sizes 0/0 and 0/1.

- Oxygen supply, tubing and related flow valves.

- Intubation equipment:

  - laryngoscopes and duplicate blades in sizes 1 and 0, spare bulbs and batteries.

  - tracheal tubes in sizes 2.5, 3.0, 3.5 and 4.0, with adapters.

  - introducers.

  - tape.

Drugs and intravenous fluids

- Intravenous access materials and cut down set.
- Adrenaline 1:10 000 solution.
- Naloxone 400 µg/ml.
- Vitamin K (Konakion®), 1 mg in 0.5 ml.
- Dextrose 10%.
- Sodium bicarbonate 4.2%. This is not generally used where basic life support is required following birth. It may be used once blood gases are available to balance an obviously unbalanced blood picture.[21] It has been suggested that if the baby has not responded to two doses of adrenaline, sodium bicarbonate will not help either.[28]
- Albumin 4.5%.
- Sodium chloride 0.9%.
- Water for injection.

Box 2.14: Resuscitation equipment available at home births[28]

- Portable suction.
- Portable oxygen.
- Bag and mask, e.g. 'Exmouth bag'.
- Good light and some form of heating.
- Torch.
- Watch or clock with a second hand.
- Notes.

---

care and the eventual inevitable transfer to the hospital. However, a good outcome can nevertheless be achieved.[21,28]

In the event of birth taking place unexpectedly and where no resuscitation equipment is available, ventilation can be carried out by the midwife covering the baby's nose and mouth with her mouth and exhaling so that the newborn's chest moves. Cardiac compression will also be necessary if the baby's heart rate is less than 60 beats per minute.

During the emergency, whether in hospital or not and despite the situation being tense and worrying, all events must be recorded accurately.

Outcomes and support

In the tension of the resuscitation situation the parents must not be forgotten. When there is silence after the delivery and the mother asks, 'is my baby all right?' it can be difficult for the midwife to know how to answer. Good communication is the key to most situations in life and most especially in this one.

Often in a hospital delivery room neither the parents nor the midwife can see what is happening at the resuscitaire or, in some cases, resuscitation is taking place outside the room. However the midwife can give the mother some idea as to what the team is doing to help the baby. The father may wish to stay with his partner or observe the resuscitation and this can only be decided with the parents at the time. Discussion after the event will also be useful for both staff and parents.

If the baby is admitted to a neonatal intensive care unit or even transferred to another hospital, the midwife should ensure that photographs are taken as soon as possible and given to the parents. They should also see the baby as soon as possible to help the attachment process.

There may be situations, particularly in preterm birth, where resuscitation has to be discontinued. Parents should be prepared by the neonatal staff as to the possible outcomes.[21,32,33,34]

The circumstances surrounding birth will affect those involved throughout their lives. Therefore it is important that doctors and midwives follow the guidelines and protocols laid down in their local practice areas to ensure they do what is right for the baby in their care.

References

1 International Liaison Committee on Resuscitation (1997) *An Advisory Statement. Resuscit.* **34**: 129–40.

2 Hayashi RH (2000) Obstetric collapse. In: L Kean, PN Baker and DI Edelstone (eds) *Best Practice in Labor Ward Management* (1e). WB Saunders, London.

3 Gregoire AS (1997) When the trauma patient is pregnant. *Regist Nurse.* **60** (2): 44–9.

4 Lee RV, Rodgers LD, White LM and Harvey AC (1986) Cardiopulmonary resuscitation of pregnant women. *Am J Med.* **81**: 311–18.

5 Stables D (1999) *Physiology in Childbearing.* Baillière Tindall, London.

6 McCunn M and Dutton R (2000) End points of resuscitation: how much is enough? *Curr Opin Anaesthesiol.* **13** (2): 147–53.

7 Blackburn ST and Loper DL (1992) *Maternal, Fetal and Neonatal Physiology: a clinical perspective.* WB Saunders, London.

8 Cox C and Grady K (1999) *Managing Obstetric Emergencies.* BIOS Scientific Publishers, Oxford.

9 Luppi CJ (1999) Cardiopulmonary resuscitation in pregnancy. *Association of Women's Health, Obstetric and Neonatal Nurses Lifelines.* **3** (3): 41–5.

10 Resuscitation Council (UK) Web site: www.nda.ox.ac.uk/rc-uk/

11 Nolan J and Gwinnutt C (1998) 1998 European guidelines on resuscitation: simplifications should make them easier to teach and implement. *BMJ.* **316** (7148): 1844–5.

12 Advanced Life Support Sub-Committee (1998) *Advanced Life Support Manual* (3e). Resuscitation Council, London.

13 Cummins R, Hazinski MD and Fran M (2000) The most important changes in the international ECC and CPR Guidelines 2000. *Circulation.* **102** (8) (Suppl): I371–6.

14 Schwalbe SS (1996) In: AV Zundert and GW Ostheimer (eds) *Pain Relief and Anaesthesia in Obstetrics.* Churchill Livingstone, London.

15 Safar P (1999) Ventilation and cardiopulmonary resuscitation. *Curr Opin Anaesthesiol.* **12** (2): 165–71.

16 Anderson MH (1997) Rhythm disorders. In: C Oakley (ed) *Heart Disease in Pregnancy.* BMJ Books, London.

17 Peerless J (2001) Fluid management of the trauma patient. *Curr Opin Anaesthesiol.* **14** (2): 221–5.

18 Williams K (1996) Witnessing resuscitation can help relatives. *Nurs Standard.* **11** (3): 12.

19 Rattrie E (2000) Witnessed resuscitation: good practice or not? *Nurs Standard.* **14** (24): 32–5.

20 Adams S (1994) Should relatives be allowed to watch resuscitation: a sister's experience. *BMJ.* **308** (6945): 1687.

21 International Liaison Committee on Resuscitation (2000) Neonatal resuscitation. *Resuscit.* **46**: 401–16.

22 Maternal and Child Health Research Consortium (2000) *Confidential Enquiry into Stillbirths and Deaths in Infancy* (Seventh Annual Report). Maternal and Child Health Research Consortium, London.

23 Department of Health (2001) NHS maternity statistics, England: 1995–96 to 1997–98. *Statistical Bulletin* **2001**: 14.

24 Johnson MH and Everitt BJ (2001) *Essential Reproduction* (5e). Blackwell Scientific, Oxford.

25 Leeson S, Edozien L and Mander T (1995) There are alternatives to Apgar. *Hosp Update.* **21** (5): 212–16.

26 Valensise H and Romanini C (1996) In: A Zundert and GW Ostheimer (eds) *Pain Relief and Anaesthesia in Obstetrics.* Churchill Livingstone, London.

27 Aynsley-Green A and Lawson GR (1990) Gut hormones and regulatory peptides in relation to enteral feeding, gastroenteritis, and necrotizing enterocolitis in infancy. *J Paediatrics.* **117** (1) (Suppl): Part 2 S24–32.

28 Drew D, Jevon P and Raby M (2000) *Resuscitation of the Newborn: a practical approach.* Butterworth Heinemann, Oxford.

29 Casey B, McIntire D and Leveno K (2001) The continuing value of the Apgar score for the assessment of newborn infants. *NEJM.* **344** (7): 467–71.

30 Hamilton P (1999) ABC of labour care: care of the newborn in the delivery room. *BMJ.* **318** (7195): 1403–6.

31 Halliday HL (2001) Endotracheal intubation at birth for preventing morbidity and mortality in vigorous, meconium-stained infants born at term. In: *The Cochrane Library*. (Issue 1). Update Software, Oxford.

32 Rennie J (1996) Perinatal management at the lower margin of viability. *Arch Dis Childhood*. **74** (3): 214–18.

33 Soll R (1999) Consensus and controversy over resuscitation of the newborn infant. *Lancet*. **354** (9172): 4–5.

34 McHaffie H (1998) Withdrawing treatment from neonates: a review of the issues. *Br J Midwif*. **6** (6): 384–8.

Further reading

- Hayman RG and Baker N (2000) Labor ward management of pre-eclampsia. In: L Kean, PN Baker and DI Edelstone (eds) *Best Practice in Labor Ward Management* (1e). WB Saunders, London.

- Reynolds F (1998) Effect of labour analgesia on the baby. *Fetal Maternal Med Rev*. **10**: 45–59.

- Richmond S and Wyllie J (2000) Newborn life support. In: *The Resuscitation Guidelines 2000*. Resuscitation Council (UK), London.

CHAPTER 3

Thromboembolism in pregnancy

Judy Bothamley

Introduction

Pulmonary thromboembolism is responsible for approximately 15 maternal deaths a year in the UK, making it the leading cause of maternal mortality in the country.[1] Pulmonary embolism (PE) occurs when a clot from a deep vein, commonly in the leg, detaches itself and travels to the lungs. Sudden death will occur if the clot is large enough to compromise the pulmonary circulation. Pregnancy is a hypercoagulable state making pregnant women more prone to developing the deep vein thrombosis (DVT) that underlies this disorder. Prevention, detection and treatment of a DVT are crucial in limiting deaths from PE in pregnancy. The management of a DVT, therefore, though not constituting an emergency of itself, will be discussed fully in this chapter alongside the immediate diagnosis and treatment of a woman presenting with a PE. Amniotic fluid embolism may present in a similar manner to a PE, or indeed be a cause of PE, but because of its extreme rarity, difficulty in diagnosis and confusion over its aetiology, it will be discussed in Chapter 7.

Epidemiology

Pregnancy is known to increase the risk of DVT and PE and yet the difficulty in diagnosing these two conditions in real life means that there is a wide range in the numbers of reported incidences

of these conditions.[2] One retrospective estimate (1990–93) of their combined incidence was 608 out of 479 422 deliveries (0.13%), consisting of 518 DVTs and 90 PEs, all confirmed by further investigations.[3] A common misconception is that DVT occurs only in late pregnancy and the postnatal period. This probably arises from the time when extended bedrest was advocated for antenatal complications and recovery during the puerperium. The use of oestrogen to suppress lactation was also formerly implicated as contributing to an increased incidence of DVT in the postnatal period. Gherman et al.'s study[4] suggested that almost 75% of DVTs occurred in the antenatal period, half of which developed before 15 weeks gestation. In the *Report on Confidential Enquiries into Maternal Deaths*,[1] 13 women died of PE in the antenatal period with eight deaths occurring in the first trimester. Epidemiological studies show that 60–70% of PEs occurred in the postpartum period with up to 82% associated with caesarean section.[4,5,6] However, PE is not common, with the overall incidence in pregnancy somewhere in the region of 0.017%.[7] In other words, a maternity unit with 5000 deliveries a year should expect to see about five women develop a confirmed DVT and perhaps a single case of PE annually.

A PE is likely to occur in 15–24% of venous thromboses that remain undiagnosed and untreated. Studies have indicated that two-thirds of deaths from pulmonary embolism occurred within 30 minutes of the embolic event.[4,6]

Pathophysiology

The risk of venous thromboembolism is five to six times higher in a pregnant woman compared to a non-pregnant woman of similar age.[2,5] Rudolf Virchow (1821–1902) first described the triad of factors that are associated with venous thrombosis, all of which are present during pregnancy (*see* Figure 3.1).[8]

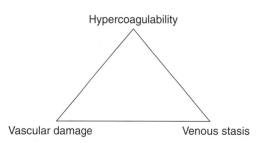

Figure 3.1 Triad of factors associated with venous thrombosis[8]

Hypercoagulability

Normal pregnancy is associated with alterations in the proteins of the coagulation and fibrinolytic systems, resulting in a relative state of hyper-coagulability.[5] These changes are an adaptive and preparatory mechanism for the control of bleeding in the third stage of labour and help maintain the placenta–uterine interface.[9] Procoagulant factors, such as von Willebrand factor, factor VIII, factor V and fibrinogen increase in pregnancy. In addition, an acquired resistance to the anticoagulant protein C and a reduction in protein S further contribute to the increased coagulability. Impaired fibrinolysis, through an increase in plasminogen activator inhibitors, also occurs.[9]

Venous stasis

Venous return from the lower limbs is reduced when the pregnant uterus compresses the inferior vena cava. Reduction of the muscle tone of veins during pregnancy, caused by progesterone, also occurs.[2,9] Blood remains in contact with the vessel wall for a longer time and this may be the most important factor in the development of a DVT.[5,10] Incompetent venous valves are a common source of morbidity in women of reproductive

age and may also contribute to venous stasis. Blood flow within the veins depends on the action of voluntary muscles and periods of inactivity further slow blood flow. The anatomy of the venous drainage from the lower limb, where the left iliac vein is crossed by the right iliac artery, means that DVTs are more common in the left leg.[9]

Vascular damage

The venous epithelium is normally an intact, smooth, single layer of cells containing various substances to prevent platelet adhesion and clot formation. Trauma damaging the vessel wall will set off a series of chemical reactions which will allow platelet aggregation at the site of injury and fibrin formation that results in the development of a clot. Increased venous distension and stasis in pregnancy may predispose to microscopically small tears in the endothelium.[10] In addition, endothelial damage to pelvic vessels can occur during vaginal or operative delivery.[9]

Additional risk factors

Of the cases documented in the last *Report on Confidential Enquiries into Maternal Deaths*, many were women who had died from complications of thrombosis having also had predisposing risk factors for thrombosis.[1] A consideration of risk factors in the context of individualised care is important in the prevention of thromboembolism. Risk assessment tools have been developed in general nursing to highlight those at risk and implement appropriate preventive measures (*see* Chapter 12 for further discussion of general issues concerning risk assessment).[8] The Royal College of Obstetricians and Gynaecologists (RCOG) has developed tools for risk assessment for women undergoing caesarean section and for those travelling by air.[11,12] Knowledge of risk factors for DVT will inform midwives in relation to care, advice and referral (*see* Box 3.1). The more important of these are discussed below.

Congenital thrombophilia

An alteration in the balance between the coagulation and fibrinolytic systems caused by congenital disorders predisposes a woman to clot

---

Box 3.1: Risk factors for venous thromboembolism in pregnancy and the postpartum period

- Caesarean section.

- Age over 35 years.

- Obesity (>80 kg) or high body mass index (BMI) (>30 kg/m^2).

- Smoking.

- Multiparity.

- Varicose veins.

- Current infection.

- Pre-eclampsia.

- Immobility, e.g. bed rest, air travel, long car journeys.

- Major current illness, e.g. heart or lung disease, cancer, inflammatory bowel disease, nephrotic syndrome.

- Major pelvic surgery.

- Personal or family history of DVT, PE or thrombophilia.

- Paralysis of the lower limbs.

- Anti-cardiolipin antibodies (antiphospholipid syndrome or as part of systemic lupus erythematosis).

- Oestrogen treatment to suppress lactation.

- Sickle-cell anaemia.

- Dehydration.

- Blood group other than O.

- Caucasian.

- Combined oral contraceptive pill.

---

formation. These include the presence of Leiden factor V (the most common cause of congenital thrombophilia), followed by deficiencies of protein C, protein S and antithrombin III. Women with known thrombophilia should be referred to a physician in early pregnancy, and preferably before conception, to discuss management options. Screening for Leiden factor V was considered in a study by Rintelen et al., when a significant number of women on the oral contraceptive pill diagnosed with a DVT or PE were found to have this mutation.[13] Screening is recommended for women with clinical features that suggest the possibility of congenital thrombophilia (*see* Box 3.2).

Previous history of thromboembolism

Not surprisingly, a previous history of thromboembolism increases the risk for thromboembolism in pregnancy probably in the region of 12–15%.[6] Women who have had a thromboembolism would normally or ideally have been screened for congenital thrombophilia prior to pregnancy.

Age over 35 years

A linear relationship between increasing age and venous thromboembolism is established in

---

Box 3.2: Features of a woman's history that suggest possible congenital thrombophilia

- Previous DVT.

- Family history of DVT.

- Recurrent and second trimester miscarriage.

- Intrauterine death.

- Severe and/or recurrent intrauterine growth restriction.

- Severe and recurrent pre-eclampsia.

Adapted from Greer.[9]

---

the general population.[14] Explanations such as the loss of elasticity of the veins may pertain to patients over 60 years of age but do not seem plausible for the relatively young age of pregnant women. Despite this, age over 35 years has been identified in a number of epidemiological studies as a significant risk factor for thromboembolism.[2,4,6] However a recent Swedish study challenges earlier findings, claiming that age as an independent variable was not significant.[3]

Multiparity

Ten per cent of women diagnosed as having venous thromboembolism had more than three children.[4] Based on analysis of maternal mortality statistics, de Swiet[2] claimed that the risk of fatal thromboembolism is 20 times greater in women over 40 years having their fifth or more pregnancy than it is in women aged 20 years in their first pregnancy.

Obesity

Obesity is an important risk factor for thromboembolism.[1,4] Data from the *Report on Confidential Enquiries into Maternal Deaths* showed that 13 of the women who died from PE were overweight.[1] This was attributed both to a susceptibility to develop a thrombosis and to inadequate anticoagulation caused by maternal weight not being

taken into account when heparin was prescribed. A body weight of over 80 kg is associated with poor mobility and an increased likelihood of venous stasis.[6] A decrease in fibrinolytic activity has also been reported in patients with a BMI greater than 25 kg/m^2.[15]

Combined oral contraception

Five of the nine late deaths reported in the *Confidential Enquiries into Maternal Deaths in the United Kingdom* were of women who had been prescribed the combined oral contraceptive pill.[1] Significantly, all these women were overweight. The risk of thromboembolism in women using oral contraception is small and well below the risk associated with pregnancy. However, *British National Formulary* guidelines do advise caution in the use of the combined oral contraceptive pill in women with other risk factors for thromboembolism, including obesity.[16]

Pre-eclampsia

Pre-eclampsia is associated with vascular injury, which in turn is related to a disturbance in coagulation, thereby suggesting a link with thromboembolism.[9] Confounding factors, such as caesarean section and bedrest, may contribute to the risk of thromboembolism in women with pre-eclampsia.

Immobility

Movement of calf muscles and deep respiratory effort promote venous return and prevent stasis. Most pregnant women are healthy and active, but there are occasions when they become less mobile and are susceptible to thromboembolism. Changes in patterns of antenatal and postnatal care have contributed to the avoidance of bedrest for pregnant women and probably account for the overall reduction in thromboembolism over the years. However, bedrest does occur after caesarean section and at a time of severe pre-eclampsia. In a recent study bedrest, as a treatment for premature labour and premature rupture of membranes, was associated with an increase in thromboembolism.[17]

The *Report on Confidential Enquiries into Maternal Deaths* reported the deaths of two pregnant women following long-haul flights and yet direct evidence for a link between venous thromboembolism and air travel in pregnant women is lacking.[1] However, studies in the non-pregnant population have raised concern about the risk and advice to all travellers on the precautionary measures for avoiding DVT is also recommended in pregnancy.[12,18,19]

The 1998 *Report on Confidential Enquiry into Maternal Deaths* reported that a paraplegic woman died of PE in the postnatal period.[20] Overcoming the problems of immobility for these women represents a particular challenge.

Caesarean section

Delivery by caesarean section increases the risk of thromboembolism by between two- and ten-fold.[3,4,21] Venous stasis, increased coagulability and vessel trauma all occur at surgery. In the 1998 *Report on Confidential Enquiries into Maternal Deaths*, 15 deaths from PE occurred following caesarean section, most of which occurred 15–28 days after surgery.[20] The last *Report on Confidential Enquiries into Maternal Deaths* showed a striking fall in deaths after caesarean section, which was attributed to the increased use of thromboprophylaxis.[1,11]

Smoking

Vessey and Doll first reported an association between cigarette smoking and DVT in 1968.[22] Nicotine was postulated to increase platelet adhesion. Lindqvist's study of 479 422 deliveries found that the smoking of more than ten cigarettes a day was significantly associated with a risk of thromboembolism.[3]

Diagnosis of deep vein thrombosis

The diagnosis of DVT in pregnancy is notoriously difficult with clinical assessment being incorrect in up to 50% of cases.[23] However, accurate diagnosis is essential, not only to prevent PE, but also to protect women from unnecessary treatment with anticoagulants. Symptoms can be helpful (*see* Box 3.3), but it is sobering to note that the

---

Box 3.3: Symptoms and signs of DVT

- Redness or discoloration of the affected leg.
- Swelling (at least 2 cm difference between the two legs).
- Leg pain or discomfort.
- Calf tenderness.
- Change in limb colour or temperature.
- Homan's sign (pain on dorsiflexion of the foot).
- Low grade fever (<37.5 C).
- Tachycardia (pulse >100/min).
- Lower abdominal pain.

---

majority of women who died from PE showed no clinical evidence of DVT.[6] General discomfort and swelling of a woman's legs in pregnancy further clouds the diagnosis. Thrombus in the pelvic veins (potentially more lethal because of their proximity to the pulmonary circulation) causes symmetrical swelling of the legs similar to the effects of the gravid uterus and is more difficult to see with ultrasonography. Referral to a senior obstetrician and careful evaluation of additional risk factors form an essential part of the clinical assessment of a woman presenting with symptoms of DVT.

Venography

This procedure has been the gold standard by which more recent developments in the diagnosis of DVT have been appraised. It involves an injection of contrast medium into the foot. Radiographic images of the leg and pelvis are examined for alterations in normal venous return.[10] Venography is an invasive procedure that is technically difficult and the contrast dye used may cause pain, swelling, redness and skin damage at the site of injection.[6] Many clinicians still advocate venography in circumstances where non-invasive studies, such as ultrasound, are equivocal.[5] It is recommended that the uterus is shielded where possible during the procedure to minimise exposure of the foetus to ionising radiation.[2,24]

Impedance plethysmography

Changes in the venous outflow in a limb are detected by this procedure of measuring changes in electrical resistance. A thigh cuff is inflated to occlude venous outflow. Release of the cuff will normally result in a rapid flow of blood. In the presence of thrombus, the rate of flow will be reduced. Impedance plethysmography is useful in pregnancy if the physiological changes, such as reduced venous tone and reduced blood flow due to the gravid uterus, are taken into account.[6] Examination, as with venography and doppler ultrasound, should take place with the woman in the left lateral position to displace the uterus from obstructing the pelvic venous flow.[5]

Ultrasonography

The use of ultrasound has now largely replaced venography for the diagnosis of DVT in maternity care. It has the advantages of being non-invasive, quick and of using standard scanning equipment available in most obstetric units.[6] Using ultrasound, the veins and thrombus can be directly seen. Doppler ultrasound, especially with a colour monitor, improves the diagnostic accuracy of this technique. When thrombus is present, a relatively echogenic soft tissue mass, which prevents the vein collapsing after compression of the leg, is seen. The vein should also become distended during a Valsalva manoeuvre, unless a clot is obstructing venous flow.[2,6] The calf veins and veins above the inguinal ligament cannot be clearly seen with this technique. Calf vein thrombosis rarely embolises, but the ultrasound examination should be repeated some days later to ensure that the thrombus has not extended into the femoral vein.[25]

Magnetic resonance imaging (MRI)

This may become the diagnostic method of choice for pelvic and ovarian vein thrombosis. The latter is a rare but serious postpartum complication, which is clinically indistinguishable from endometritis, appendicitis or pyelonephritis; ovarian vein thrombosis may cause sepsis or PE.[26]

Fibrin degradation products (D-dimer)

D-dimers are formed as a thrombus develops and can be measured in the blood to raise suspicion of a DVT. D-dimer assays are commonly used in conjunction with ultrasound in non-pregnant patients. However, false positives are common, especially in pregnancy and are of no clinical value in the postpartum period. Low levels of D-dimer in pregnancy are likely, as in non-pregnant patients, to suggest that there is no thrombus.[23]

Diagnosis of pulmonary embolism

The clinical signs of PE are related to the size of the clot that is obstructing the pulmonary circulation. Large or multiple emboli will prevent adequate oxygenation of the blood and may even reduce the cardiac output due to poor venous return from the systemic and pulmonary circulations.[6,10] A woman with a major PE will collapse with hypotension, chest pain and occasionally abdominal pain, breathlessness and cyanosis. On closer examination a third heart sound, parasternal heave and an elevated jugular venous pressure may be present. Sudden respiratory or cardiac arrest may occur. The identification of a major PE is usually obvious, but many symptoms of an acute minor embolism, which may warn of an impending fatal embolus, are non-specific and similar to other cardiopulmonary diseases (see Box 3.4). Warning signs and symptoms indicative of smaller emboli include unexplained pyrexia, cough, chest pain and breathlessness, which may be incorrectly diagnosed as a chest infection. An infective cause for these symptoms should only be considered after a PE has been excluded. Breathlessness, rapid breathing and leg discomfort occur commonly as pregnancy progresses and consequently might be ignored. Signs and symptoms associated with minor PE are listed in Box 3.5. Any of these, in combination with a DVT, would indicate the need for treatment.

A chest x-ray, electrocardiogram (ECG) and oxygen levels (saturation and blood gases) will not confirm the diagnosis, but will help build a picture of the woman's condition and identify other aetiologies. With a PE the chest x-ray may

---

Box 3.4: Differential diagnosis in PE

- Chest infection.
- Pneumothorax.
- Pulmonary aspiration.
- Amniotic fluid embolism.
- Intra-abdominal bleeding.
- Septicaemia.
- Intracerebral haemorrhage.
- Hypo- and hyperglycaemia.
- Aortic aneurysm.
- Myocardial infarction.

Box 3.5: Clinical manifestations of PE

Most frequent signs and symptoms

- Breathlessness.
- Pleuritic chest pain.
- Cough.
- Peripheral oedema.
- Crackles on listening to the chest.

Associated signs and symptoms

- Haemoptysis.
- Tachypnoea.
- Tachycardia.
- Hypertension.
- Distended neck veins.
- Cyanosis.
- Tricuspid flow murmur.
- Acute cor pulmonale.
- Anxiety.
- Fever.

be initially normal, although non-specific abnormalities, such as atelectasis, unilateral pleural effusion, areas of consolidation or elevation of the hemidiaphragm may be seen as the PE causes areas of infarction and inflammation in the lung tissue.[27] The chest x-ray findings are important in clarifying the interpretation of the ventilation-perfusion scan (V/Q scan). The ECG can show right heart strain or right bundle branch block; the former can be found during pregnancy and the latter can be a normal finding. Hypoxia at rest or a fall in oxygen saturation on exercise with a pulse oximeter is not specific, but increases the likelihood of a PE. Arterial gases, if taken, should be carried out with the woman in an upright position. Blood gases may be normal in approximately 10% of patients with PE,[10] although hypoxaemia and primary respiratory alkalosis in the absence of other pulmonary disease is most likely to be due to PE.[2,10]

A V/Q scan is the most useful diagnostic test for PE. The perfusion component of the scan involves intravenous injection of albumin labelled with radioactive technetium. The distribution of the pulmonary blood flow is assessed and segmental areas with reduced or absent perfusion are diagnostic of PE.[10] The radiation dose is low, below that which is known to be harmful to the foetus.[2] The ventilation component of the V/Q scan increases the sensitivity of identifying under-perfused and under-ventilated areas by collecting information regarding the distribution of inhaled gas. PE typically produces poor perfusion in an area of normal ventilation.[10] If ventilation as well as perfusion is reduced, the condition is likely to be infective.[2]

Treatment

Anticoagulation

Once thromboembolism is diagnosed in pregnancy, rapid and prolonged anticoagulation is required to prevent extension of the thrombus, restore venous patency and limit the risk or recurrence of a PE.[27] The aim of treatment in the acute phase is to produce as high an anticoagulation as possible without putting the woman at risk of spontaneous bleeding.[2]

Unfractionated heparin (UH)

The most widely prescribed and effective anticoagulant used in pregnancy has traditionally been UH. Heparin is a large molecule that does not cross the placenta, so the risk of teratogenesis or bleeding in the foetus is minimal. It is therefore considered safe for use during pregnancy and lactation.[6,10,28]

Heparin works by binding to and accelerating the activity of anti-thrombin III, a protein that inhibits activated factor X (Xa). Inhibition of factor Xa is important in preventing the formation of thrombin.[29] Heparin is thought not to facilitate the breakdown of thrombus but to act to prevent further propagation of clot formation.[2] Different regimens exist for acute treatment of thromboembolism in pregnancy using heparin (see Box 3.6 for a summary of a typical approach) and midwives should familiarise themselves with local guidelines. Any regime needs to be supported by appropriate monitoring to quickly establish and maintain therapeutic levels (see Table 3.1). Prior to treatment with heparin, blood should be taken for a full blood count (including platelets), activated partial thromboplastin time (APTT) and prothrombin time (PT);[27] de Swiet also recommends routine screening for antithrombin III deficiency.[21] APTT monitoring can be technically difficult particularly in late pregnancy when an apparent heparin resistance occurs. This can lead to unnecessarily high doses of heparin being used with subsequent risk of haemorrhage.[23] Heparin is cleared by the kidney so that caution should be exercised in women with renal impairment or pre-eclampsia.[6] Heparin-induced thrombocytopaenia is rare, but the platelet count should be rechecked at 5–14 days after the start of heparin therapy and monthly thereafter.[24,28] Long-term heparin therapy with doses of 10 000 IU for up to ten months is associated with osteoporosis.[6,30,31] Pregnancy and breast-feeding themselves cause reversible bone demineralisation, which may exacerbate the problem.[24] A few cases of vertebral fractures have occurred in women on long-term heparin therapy.[31] The use of low molecular weight heparin and/or switching to warfarin postnatally provides an alternative, otherwise the risk of thromboembolism has to be balanced against the potential risk of fracture.[24]

Low molecular weight heparin (LMWH)

The last ten years have seen the development of LMWH. There are several LMWHs, but the most commonly used in pregnancy are enoxaparin (Clexane®) and dalteparin (Fragmin®).[21,32] LMWH is formed by the enzymatic depolymerisation of unfractionated heparin yielding smaller molecules.[29] All heparins exert their effect by binding to

---

Box 3.6: Treatment of minor thromboembolism in pregnancy[5,21,27]

At presentation

- Unfractionated heparin as a bolus 5000–10 000 IU intravenously (IV) followed by continuous infusion of 1000–1600 IU per hour for 5–10 days.

Maintenance

- 10 000 IU unfractionated heparin twice a day (b.d.) or low molecular weight heparin subcutaneously, dose according to body weight.

In labour

- Heparin 7500 IU b.d. subcutaneously or continue low molecular weight heparin (epidural block or instrumental delivery are not contraindicated if thrombin time and activated partial thromboplastin time is normal).

Postpartum

- Continue heparin at 7500 IU b.d. subcutaneously then heparin or warfarin for at least five weeks.

Table 3.1: Laboratory tests for monitoring heparin therapy[27]

Assay	Nature of the test	Therapeutic range	Comments
Activated partial thromboplastin time (APTT)	Measures time to clot formation after adding an activating agent	Double the control	Can be difficult to measure and unpredictable in pregnancy
Protamine titration	Determines the plasma level of heparin	0.2–0.4 U/ml	
Thrombin time (TT)	Thrombin is added to the plasma and time to clot recorded	Maintenance – not prolonged	
Anti-factor Xa assay	Measures the rate of factor Xa inhibition by optical density determination	0.8–1.0 U/ml acutely; <0.2 U/ml maintenance	Expensive; low molecular weight heparin (LMWH) – specific; not widely available

antithrombin III and potentiating the inhibition of factor Xa. LMWH has a decreased affinity for thrombin;[32] its increased bioavailability and longer half-life, compared to standard preparations, permits once daily administration, an obvious benefit for women on long-term anticoagulant therapy.[21] Several clinical trials have supported the superior efficacy and relative safety of LMWH both in pregnant and non-pregnant populations.[33,34] LMWH has a more predictable response so that laboratory monitoring is rarely required. There is also a less frequent incidence of heparin-induced thrombocytopaenia and osteopaenia.[29] LMWH does not appear to cross the placenta or enter the foetal circulation and major risk of bleeding in the mother seems less.[32,34,35] With such positive benefits, LMWH is commonly used for prophylaxis of thromboembolism and for the chronic phase of treatment, and is now replacing the use of unfractionated or standard heparin.[23,36,37]

The therapeutic dose of LMWHs are maternal weight dependent and failure to achieve adequate anticoagulation was thought in the *Report on Confidential Enquiries into Maternal Deaths* to have been a factor in the death of one obese woman.[1] The RCOG has issued guidelines on the dosage of enoxaparin in relation to early pregnancy weight.[23] In the light of their experience Thompson et al.[36] recommend that LMWH may also be useful for the treatment of acute thromboembolism in pregnancy; however evidence to support the use of LMWH in acute situations is limited. Concerns over dosage and risk of bleeding during labour and the potential for spinal haematoma when an epidural is sited or removed remain. Measurement of anti-Xa activity may be helpful in monitoring therapeutic

activity in these circumstances.[33,38,39] Spinal haematoma is a rare, but serious, complication of epidural anaesthesia that may cause permanent neurological damage. Women receiving heparin therapy prior to regional block should have their coagulation screen checked before the insertion of an epidural catheter.[6] Midwives should note anaesthetists' instructions and hospital policy regarding the timing of removal of an epidural catheter.

Warfarin

An oral anticoagulant with a small molecule, warfarin readily crosses the placenta. As a known teratogen, it is not commonly used in pregnancy. The foetus is particularly vulnerable between six and 12 weeks' gestation, although the central nervous system abnormalities associated with warfarin use have been reported throughout pregnancy. However, warfarin is considered safe during lactation. Warfarin is started three days prior to stopping heparin. The international normalised ratio (INR) of prothrombin time is used to measure warfarin's anticoagulant effect. The need for regular venepuncture to check the INR during treatment may negate the benefits of an oral anticoagulant.[6]

Emergency resuscitation and the management of life-threatening pulmonary embolism

Two-thirds of deaths caused by PE are estimated to occur within the first hour following an embolic event and the remainder within four to six hours.[40] Early diagnosis and treatment represent an important clinical challenge for the multidisciplinary team. In the UK at present most women with this condition are likely to be cared for in an intensive care unit, but with the increased introduction of high dependency units in maternity areas, the midwife could become involved. This section therefore discusses emergency resuscitation with detail of the midwifery role and responsibilities and the various medical interventions that may be pursued to prevent death from PE.

A woman presenting with massive pulmonary embolus will suffer cardiovascular collapse. If conscious, she is likely to be cyanotic, breathless and complaining of pain in her chest or shoulders. Appropriate staff, including a senior anaesthetist and physician, should be urgently summoned to deal with this emergency or if the woman is at home, she should be immediately transferred to the closest accident and emergency department via ambulance. The surgical team and a radiologist will also be required.

Immediate treatment should be standard assessment and appropriate cardiac arrest procedure (*see* Chapter 2). Prolonged cardiac massage is recommended as it is thought this may break up the original clot and permit an increase in pulmonary blood flow.[2]

If the woman is making some respiratory effort it is advisable to put the head of the bed up by 30 degrees and give oxygen via nasal prongs or face mask to minimise dyspnoea and attempt to improve oxygen saturation. Endotracheal intubation and mechanical ventilation may be required. If the cause of the collapse is thought likely to be PE, intravenous heparin should be given.[23] The midwife should provide the necessary support to the anaesthetist and/or physician in instigating these therapies.

Other specific midwifery management includes the assessment and documentation of respiratory and cardiovascular vital signs. Assessment of oxygen saturation levels will be made initially with an oximeter and then via arterial blood gas monitoring. An electrocardiograph (ECG) recording will be needed. Intravenous access will have been established as soon as possible. Accurate recording of fluid balance, including hourly urine output after catheterisation, is important in preventing further insult to the cardiovascular system through fluid overload: a central venous pressure (CVP) or arterial line may be necessary.

The woman, if conscious, will be extremely apprehensive and agitated. A calm, confident, sympathetic approach by the midwife may help to minimise this apprehension. A small dose of intravenous opiate (1–2 mg morphine) is recommended by some to help reduce discomfort and apprehension as well as reduce systemic afterload.[10] Members of the woman's family will require support, guidance and information at the time and following this event. Midwifery staff may also need to take responsibility for the care of the newborn. Box 3.7 summarises the main responsibilities for the midwife, a number of which can be instigated in the home setting whilst emergency transfer to hospital is arranged.

Box 3.7: Midwife's responsibilities in pulmonary embolism emergency

- Summon the emergency response team or arrange emergency transfer to hospital.

- Summon the appropriate senior staff.

- Administer cardiac massage as necessary.

- Give oxygen via nasal prongs or mask.

- Initiate IV access.

- If appropriate, sit the woman up to maximise respiratory effort.

- Assist with endotracheal intubation as necessary.

- Assess and record cardiovascular and respiratory vital signs.

- Attach oximeter and record ECG.

- Give heparin and other drugs according to medical orders.

- Maintain accurate fluid balance.

- Monitor foetal well-being as appropriate.

- Support the woman and her family.

Medical or surgical interventions in life-threatening pulmonary embolism

Thrombolytic therapy

Thrombolytic drugs are only used for treatment of PE where there is a large clot, profound hypoxia and significant circulatory collapse.[10] Three thrombolytic agents, streptokinase, urokinase and recombinant tissue plasminogen activator (rt-PA), have been used for the treatment of such life-threatening PE.[10] These drugs act to break up a clot by activating plasminogen to form plasma which degrades the fibrin in the clot.[16] However, their use, particularly in pregnancy, is problematic due to the risk of major haemorrhage. The risk of placental abruption and foetal death is unknown.[27] Bleeding from the placental site or any surgical wounds is a real concern if employed around the time of delivery or the early puerperium.[6] Thrombolytic therapy is usually given intravenously, but for a more specific action can be put directly into the pulmonary artery through the catheter used for pulmonary arteriogram.[10] Streptokinase was the first thrombolytic agent used for the treatment of PE in non-pregnant patients, but urokinase and rt-PA are thought to work more rapidly. Streptokinase is also more likely to cause anaphylaxis. rt-PA has a more specific action and therefore bleeding complications, although still constituting a major risk, may be reduced when compared with the use of urokinase and streptokinase. The evidence for the use of rt-PA in pregnancy is limited to case study reports at this stage.[39]

Inferior vena cava filters

Inferior vena cava filters have been used safely and effectively in pregnancy. Filters function by intercepting emboli travelling to the pulmonary vasculature and are used in cases where recurring clots are developing despite adequate anticoagulation and when clot extension into the common iliac vein or inferior vena cava occurs.[6,40]

Pulmonary embolectomy

Pulmonary embolectomy is rarely used to treat PE. It is a technically difficult procedure involving circulatory standstill or cardiopulmonary bypass.[21] Most patients will die before they can be transported to the appropriate surgical facility.[10] However, Woodward et al.[41] describe the successful pulmonary embolectomy on a patient who was undergoing caesarean section in a unit where cardiothoracic and obstetric facilities existed on the same site. Pulmonary angiography is carried out prior to embolectomy to locate the embolus. It may be possible to break up the clot using a guideline wire via a cardiac catheter at this time and thus avoid pulmonary embolectomy.[2,42]

Midwifery management of deep vein thrombosis

Bedrest or ambulation

Bedrest for treatment of DVT remains a dilemma. Bedrest may prevent propagation of the clot, but conversely may contribute to its further development.[10] Whilst the evidence is minimal it would seem that women should be encouraged to mobilise once anticoagulants have been started and they have been fitted with compression stockings.[23,42,43]

Leg elevation

Non-pregnant patients with DVT are advised to elevate the leg 10–20 degrees above the level of the heart to enhance venous return and reduce swelling.[10] However, in the pregnant woman inguinal congestion may occur in this position due to the enlarged uterus impeding venous return. Compression to the popliteal space behind the knee should also be avoided. Pregnant women with a DVT should find a comfortable position when in bed, perhaps with the affected leg supported along its entire length by pillows. When mobile, they should avoid standing still for long periods and when sitting should have their legs elevated.

Thromboembolic deterrant (TED) or compression stockings

Compression stockings promote venous return and decrease leg swelling.[10] External compression increases the velocity of blood flow within the veins reducing venous stasis. The risk of a clot forming is minimised by the prevention of venous wall distension and a reduction in local contact time. In addition valvular insufficiency is improved when compression stockings are worn.[44] Graduated compression stockings where compression is graduated at the ankle and decreases proximally have been demonstrated to improve blood flow and are therefore favoured.[44] Graduated compression stockings have been shown to prevent primary and recurrent DVT. For example, a significant reduction in venous thrombosis was shown when stockings were used prophylactically in patients undergoing gynaecological surgery.[45] Whilst clinical data on the effect of stockings in preventing DVT in pregnancy is lacking, evidence of an improvement in venous haemodynamics of the legs during pregnancy and the postpartum period has been shown.[44,46] It seems reasonable that the benefits shown in non-pregnant individuals would also apply in pregnancy. The use of compression stockings in the management of DVT is to decrease the risk and severity of post-thrombotic syndrome, a condition probably caused by damage to venous valves.[44] Post-thrombotic syndrome varies from mild oedema to incapacitating swelling with pain and ulceration. Early application of compression stockings in patients and pregnant women with acute DVT may prevent this complication by stimulating the development of collateral circulation and increasing fibrinolytic activity.[47,48]

Direct evidence of the value of graduated compression stockings in preventing fatal PE is inconclusive due to the difficulty in getting a sample large enough to show a significant reduction in such a relatively rare event.[44]

Accurate fitting of stockings may be more difficult in pregnancy due to changing levels of oedema. Agu et al.[44] in their review of the evidence comparing knee-length to thigh-length stockings, concluded that knee-length stockings should be used as they were equally effective, cheaper, more likely to fit correctly and better tolerated by the people wearing them.

Education, advice and support for women on anticoagulant treatment

Women generally show initial reluctance to giving themselves heparin injections and the midwife should work through the requirements with the woman to develop her confidence. A clear incentive to achieving self management will be the possibility of discharge from hospital. Heparin, either unfractionated or LMW, involves only small volumes given with a fine gauge needle. The site of subcutaneous injection should rotate between thighs and abdominal wall. Grasping some flesh, the injection is made at right angles to the skin surface. Arrangements for safe disposal of needles should be made. Bruising inevitably occurs at the site of injection. The woman should take care to take precautions in situations that may cause bleeding or injury; for example, a soft bristle toothbrush will protect from bleeding gums.[49]

A phone call or visit from the midwife within days of discharge from hospital may be timely to offer support to the woman as she comes to terms with what will be prolonged treatment. A discussion regarding the management of any future pregnancies should be made at an appropriate time, probably after delivery, and in conjunction with the physician. The woman's risk of recurrent DVT, use of the combined contraceptive pill and the potential need for anticoagulant prophylaxis in future pregnancies should be discussed.

Thromboprophylaxis in pregnancy and the puerperium

Thromboprophylaxis during pregnancy for women at increased risk of thromboembolism is an important area in preventing deaths from PE. A reduction in deaths following caesarian delivery has been attributed to thromboprophylaxis.[1] In addition, women who have experienced a thromboembolic event will require information regarding the risk of recurrence and the need for thromboprophylaxis during subsequent pregnancies. The prevention of DVT for pregnant women travelling by air is now given higher profile.[12]

Prophylaxis for pregnant women with a history of thromboembolism

In their review of the literature Toglia and Weg[5] suggest that the recurrence of a thrombosis during a subsequent pregnancy is in the region of 4–15%. However, concerns about demineralisation of bone and other maternal side effects of long-term heparin therapy, along with the lack of prospective data, have led physicians to debate the merits, or otherwise, of heparin prophylaxis throughout pregnancy and thus firm clinical guidelines have not been established.[5,9,21]

De Swiet, considered to have substantial experience in this area, recommends treatment regimens based on whether women are considered high or low risk.[21] Women with low risk of recurrence of thromboembolism (according to his definition) are those who have had one previous episode of thromboembolism only, with no additional risk factors such as thrombophilia or a family history of thromboembolism which may indicate as yet undiagnosed congenital thrombophilia. According to de Swiet, a previous DVT in pregnancy or whilst taking the oral combined contraceptive pill does not make recurrence in pregnancy any more likely than thromboembolism occurring under other circumstances.[21] Treatment for low-risk women avoids long-term heparin therapy by recommending a daily dose of aspirin 75 mg from the time of antenatal booking, heparin during and for one week following delivery and then heparin or warfarin for a further five weeks. The rationale for de Swiet's approach is based on the effectiveness of low dose aspirin in prevention of thromboembolism in surgical and medical patients and the known relative safety for use of aspirin in pregnancy established during the CLASP trial.[50,51] This conservative approach needs to be discussed fully with the woman. Her previous experience of thromboembolism, her knowledge of the side effects, her feelings about heparin therapy and her perspective of her risk of recurrence will have a bearing on the management she chooses.

Women considered to be at high risk are those who have had multiple thromboembolic episodes, thrombophilia or a family history of thrombo-embolism. Women with a deficiency of anti-thrombin III, for example, have a 70% incidence of thrombosis during pregnancy.[5] Consequently women with known or suspected thrombophilia should be referred to a unit that specialises in the management of this condition in pregnancy. They should receive heparin prophylaxis (usually LMWH) from booking.[21] Greer[9] makes similar recommendations although the gestation at which he suggests commencing heparin therapy varies according to the woman's history and he argues that prophylaxis may need to be extended to three months postpartum in some women with severe thrombotic problems. He also recommends the use of graduated compression stockings to be included in all regimens of prophylaxis.

Prophylaxis for women delivered by caesarean section

Delivery by caesarean section increases the risk of thromboembolism significantly (see above). RCOG guidelines using risk assessment to guide the use of prophylaxis at the time of caesarean delivery have been widely adopted in the UK (see Box 3.8).[11] Early mobilisation and hydration should be started in all women after caesarean delivery and is considered adequate prophylaxis for those at low risk. Deep breathing should also be encouraged in the postoperative period. Women assessed as being at moderate risk should receive either heparin prophylaxis or wear graduated compression stockings. Women in the high-risk category are advised to wear stockings in addition to heparin prophylaxis.

External pneumatic compression boots are used in some units during surgery. They are thought to reduce the development of a DVT by applying intermittent pressure to the lower limbs thus augmenting the calf muscle action that promotes venous return.[10]

Prophylaxis for pregnant women travelling by air

Precautionary measures to avoid DVT are recommended for pregnant women travelling by air. These include leg and ankle exercises, walking around the cabin when possible and avoiding dehydration by drinking plenty of non-alcoholic drinks and by minimising alcohol and caffeine intake. Other measures, including the wearing of compression stockings, LMWH prophylaxis

---

Box 3.8: Risk assessment profile for thromboembolism in caesarean section

Low risk: early mobilisation and hydration

- Elective caesarean section, uncomplicated pregnancy and no other risk factors.

Moderate risk: consider one of a variety of prophylactic measures

- Age (>35 yrs).

- Obesity (>80 kg).

- Parity four or more.

- Gross varicose veins.

- Current infection.

- Pre-eclampsia.

- Immobility prior to surgery (>4 days).

- Major current illness, e.g. heart or lung disease, cancer, inflammatory bowel disease, nephrotic syndrome.

- Emergency caesarean section in labour.

High risk: heparin prophylaxis with or without leg stockings

- Three or more moderate risk factors from above.

- Extended major pelvic or abdominal surgery, e.g. caesarean hysterectomy.

- Personal or family history of deep vein thrombosis, pulmonary embolism or thrombophilia, or paralysis of the lower limbs.

- Presence of antiphospholipid antibody (cardiolipin antibody or lupus anticoagulant).

Reproduced with permission of RCOG.[11]

---

and the use of low dose asprin, are advocated according to risk factors and the length of the flight.[12]

Midwifery responsibilities

The midwife should ask the woman about any family or personal history of thromboembolism when recording an antenatal booking history. Risk factors (*see* Box 3.1) for thromboembolism should be documented. The *Report on Confidential Enquiries into Maternal Deaths* recommends that the BMI is calculated on all women to identify those who are over 30 kg/m².[1] The identification of women with possible congenital thrombophilia (*see* Box 3.2) should be made in order that screening tests can be performed, although ideally

this would have been done before conception. The referral of women with congenital thrombophilia to a specialised unit is recommended. Health promotion strategies may be used to address issues such as smoking and obesity.[49] A plan of care should be identified in conjunction with the woman and with the multidisciplinary team for women with existing medical conditions and other risk factors such as paraplegia. The midwife and the woman can discuss strategies for prevention of thromboembolism based on the woman's history, circumstances and predisposing factors.

During subsequent antenatal visits, risk factors arising during the course of the pregnancy should be identified (*see* Box 3.1). The need for hospitalisation will increase the risk of thromboembolism and timely education about leg exercises, regular fluid intake and correct sitting position may be beneficial. The need for heparin prophylaxis and compression stockings should be discussed with the obstetrician or physician when multiple risk factors are present in women requiring prolonged hospitalisation. Regimens for thromboprophylaxis in relation to caesarean delivery, air travel and vaginal delivery should be noted and implemented.

The midwife may examine the woman's legs during each clinical assessment noting the size, colour and any temperature difference between the limbs. Homan's sign can be used, but it is more important for the midwife to listen to the woman when she is describing symptoms and put these in context. Any signs and symptoms of DVT or possible minor PE should be referred immediately to medical staff and diagnosis actively pursued.

As pregnancy itself increases a woman's risk of developing a DVT, midwives should give information to all pregnant women on ways to prevent venous stasis and promote venous return. Regular exercise such as walking and drinking adequate fluids will help. Pregnant women should avoid sitting with their legs crossed or standing for prolonged periods of time and may find it helpful to put their legs up when sitting down. They should avoid long car journeys without stopping to move around. If in a train or plane, they should walk around and do leg exercises, including ankle flexion and extension. Wearing support stockings will not only prevent feelings of tiredness and strain on the legs but may also work to prevent varicose veins. Some women will be advised to wear TED stockings. Pregnant women should avoid wearing constrictive garments around their legs and pelvic area.

Conclusions

Regimes for thromboprophylaxis in pregnancy have not been evaluated in clinical trials and debate continues in many areas, including whether or not all women having a caesarean section should receive some form of specific anti-thrombotic treatment.[21] With the rising number of caesarean deliveries being performed, there is a need for evidence from randomised controlled trials to evaluate the efficacy and safety of routine thromboprophylaxis with heparin. Guidelines are also being developed for the management of women with risk factors for thromboembolism following vaginal delivery.[1,9]

Detection of thromboembolism in pregnancy is essential in preventing deaths from PE.[1] Midwives need to be alert to the signs and symptoms of DVT, particularly in those with additional risk factors, and make appropriate referral. Prevention of thromboembolism in pregnancy includes the use of effective prophylactic measures and client education.

As in any emergency situation, if a woman collapses with a major PE, the midwife must implement appropriate resuscitation procedures immediately.

References

1 Lewis G (ed) (2001) *Why Mothers Die 1997–1999: the fifth report of the confidential enquiries into maternal deaths in the United Kingdom.* RCOG Press, London.

2 De Swiet M (1995) Thromboembolism. In: M de Swiet (ed) *Medical Disorders in Obstetric Practice* (3e). Blackwell Science, Oxford.

3 Lindqvist P, Dahlback B and Marsal K (1999) Thrombotic risk during pregnancy: a population study. *Obstet Gynecol.* **94**: 595–9.

4 Gherman RB, Goodwin M, Leung B, Byrne JD, Hethumani R and Montoro M (1999) Incidence, clinical characteristics and timing of objectively diagnosed venous thromboembolism during pregnancy. *Obstet Gynecol.* **94**: 730–4.

5 Toglia MR and Weg JG (1996) Current concepts: venous thromboembolism during pregnancy. *NEJM.* **335**: 108–14.

6 Greer IA (1996) The special case of venous thromboembolism in pregnancy. In: JE Tooke and GDO Lowe (eds) *A Textbook of Vascular Medicine.* Arnold, London.

7 Rutherford S, Montoro M, McGhee W and Strong T (1991) Thromboembolic disease associated with pregnancy: an 11-year review. *Am J Obstet Gynecol.* **164** (Suppl): 286.

8 Autar R (1996) *Deep Vein Thrombosis: the silent killer.* Quay Books, Dinton.

9 Greer IA (1999) Thrombosis in pregnancy: maternal and fetal issues. *Lancet.* **353**: 1258–65.

10 Walsh ME and Rice KL (1999) Venous thrombosis and pulmonary embolism. In: VA Fahey (ed) *Vascular Nursing* (3e). WB Saunders, London.

11 Royal College of Obstetricians and Gynaecologists Working Party (1995) *Prophylaxis*

against Thromboembolism in Gynaecology and Obstetrics. RCOG Press, London.

12 Royal College of Obstetricians and Gynaecologists Scientific Advisory Committee (2001) *Advice on Preventing Deep Vein Thrombosis for Pregnant Women Travelling by Air* (Opinion Paper 1). RCOG Press, London.

13 Rintelen C, Mannhalter C, Ireland H, Lane DA, Knobl P, Lechner K and Pabinger I (1996) Oral contraceptives enhance the risk of clinical manifestations of venous thrombosis at a young age in females homozygous for factor V Leiden. *Br J Haematol.* **93**: 487–90.

14 Office of Population Censuses and Surveys (1999). *Mortality Statistics Cause: England and Wales I.* A publication of the government statistical services. The Stationery Office, London.

15 Pollen L (1993) *Recent Advances in Blood Coagulation* (Vol 6). Churchill Livingstone, Edinburgh.

16 British Medical Association and the Royal Pharmaceutical Society of Great Britain (1999) *British National Formulary.* **Sept**: 117.

17 Kovacevich GJ, Gaich SA, Lavin JP, Hopkins MP, Crane SS, Stewart J, Nelson D and Lavin LM (2000). The prevalence of thromboembolic events among women with extended bed rest prescribed as part of the treatment for premature labor or preterm premature rupture of membranes. *Am J Obstet Gynecol.* **182**: 1089–92.

18 Hirsh J and O'Donnell MJ (2001) Venous thromboembolism after long flights: are airlines to blame? *Lancet.* **357**: 1461–2.

19 Scurr JH, Machin SJ, Bailey-King S, Mackie IJ, McDonald S and Smith PDC (2001) Frequency and prevention of symptomless deep-vein thrombosis in long-haul flights: a randomised trial. *Lancet.* **357**: 1485–9.

20 Department of Health (1998) *Why Mothers Die: report on confidential enquiry into maternal deaths in the United Kingdom 1994–1996.* The Stationery Office, London.

21 De Swiet M (1999) Thromboembolic disease. In: D James, P Steer, C Weiner and B Gonik (eds) *High Risk Pregnancy: management options.* WB Saunders, London.

22 Vessey MP and Doll R (1968) Investigation of the relation between use of oral contraceptives and thromboembolic disease. *BMJ.* **2**: 199–205.

23 Royal College of Obstetrics and Gynaecologists (2001) *Thromboembolic Disease in Pregnancy and the Puerperium*: acute management (Guideline 28). RCOG Press, London.

24 Nelson-Piercy C (1997) *Handbook of Obstetric Medicine.* Isis Medical Media, Oxford.

25 Rutherford SE and Phelan JP (1991) Deep vein thrombosis and pulmonary embolism in pregnancy. *Obstet Gynecol Clin N Am.* **18**: 345–70.

26 Hippach M, Meyberg R, Villena-Heinson C, Mink D, Ertan AK, Scmidt W and Friedrich M (2000) Postpartum ovarian vein thrombosis. *Clin Exp Obstet Gynecol.* **27**: 24–6.

27 Toglia MR and Nolan TE (1997) Venous thromboembolism during pregnancy: a current review of diagnosis and management. *Obstet Gynecol Surv.* **52**: 60–72.

28 Barbour LA and Pickard J (1995) Controversies in thromboembolic disease during pregnancy: a critical review. *Obstet Gynecol.* **86**: 621–33.

29 Aguilar D and Goldhaber SZ (1999) Clinical uses of low molecular weight heparins. *Chest.* **115**: 1418–23.

30 Ginsberg JS (1996) Drug therapy: management of venous thromboembolism. *NEJM.* **335**: 1816–28.

31 Dahlman T, Lindvall N and Hellgren M (1990) Osteopenia in pregnancy during long-term heparin treatment: a radiological study post partum. *Br J Obstet Gynaecol.* **97**: 221–8.

32 Chan WS and Ray JG (1999) Low molecular weight heparin use during pregnancy: issues of safety and practicality. *Obstet Gynecol Surv.* **54**: 649–54.

33 Duplaga BA, Rivers CW and Nutescu E (2001) Dosing and monitoring of low-molecular-weight heparin in special populations. *Pharmacotherapy.* **21**: 218–34.

34 Ginsberg JS, Greer I and Hirsh J (2001) Use of antithrombotic agents during pregnancy. *Chest.* **119** (Supp 1): 122–31.

35 Ellison J, Walker ID and Greer IA (2000) Antenatal use of enoxaparin for prevention and treatment of thromboembolism in pregnancy. *Br J Obstet Gynecol.* **107**: 1116–21.

36 Thompson AJ, Walker ID and Greer IA (1998) Low-molecular-weight heparin for immediate management of thromboembolic disease in pregnancy. *Lancet.* **352**: 1904.

37 Greer IA (2001) Treatment of venous thromboembolism in pregnancy. *Repro Vasc Med.* **1**: 114–23.

38 Tam WH, Wong KS, Yuen PM, Leung TN and Li CY (1999) Low-molecular-weight heparin and thromboembolism in pregnancy. *Lancet.* **353**: 932.

39 Narayan H, Culliman J, Karup K et al. (1992) Experience with the cardial inferior vena cava filter as prophylaxis against pulmonary embolism in pregnant women with extensive deep vein thrombosis. *Br J Obstet Gynaecol.* **99**: 726.

40 Nishimura K, Kawaguchi M, Shimokawa M, Kitaguchi K and Furuya H (1998) Treatment of pulmonary embolism during caesarean section with recombinant plasminogen activator. *Anesthesiol.* **89**: 1027–8.

41 Woodward DK, Birks RJ and Granger KA (1999) Massive pulmonary embolism in late pregnancy. *Can J Anaesthetics.* **46**: 906.

42 Partsch H and Blattler W (2000) Compression and walking versus bed rest in the management of proximal deep vein thrombosis with low molecular weight heparin. *J Vasc Surg.* **35**: 861–9.

43 Manganaro A, Buda D, Calabro D, Tati L and Consolo F (2000) Physical treatment of deep vein thrombosis. *Minerva Cardioangiol.* **48**: 53–6.

44 Agu O, Hamilton G and Baker D (1999) Graduated compression stockings in the prevention of venous thromboembolism. *Br J Surg.* **86**: 992–1004.

45 Turner GM, Cole SE and Brooks JH (1984) The efficacy of graduated compression stockings in the prevention of deep vein thrombosis after major gynaecological surgery. *Br J Obstet Gynaecol.* **91**: 588–91.

46 Buchtemann AS, Steins A, Volkert B, Hahn M, Klyscz T and Junger M (1999) The effect of compression therapy on venous haemodynamics in pregnant women. *Br J Obstet Gynaecol.* **106**: 563–9.

47 Lowe GD (1997) Treatment of venous thrombo-embolism. *Baillières Clin Obstet Gynaecol.* **11**: 511–21.

48 Brandjes DPM, Buller HR, Heijboer H, Huisman MV, de Rijk M, Jagt H and ten Cate JW (1997) Randomised trial of compression stockings in patients with symptomatic proximal-vein thrombosis. *Lancet.* **349**: 759–62.

49 Bewley C and Bradshaw C (2001) Thromboembolic disorders during pregnancy, birth and the puerperium. *MIDIRS Midwif Digest.* **11**: 56–9.

50 Antiplatelet Trialist Collaboration (1994) Collaborative overview of randomised trials of antiplatelet therapy (III): reduction in venous thrombosis and pulmonary embolism by antiplatelet prophylaxis among surgical and medical patients. *BMJ.* **308**: 235–46.

51 CLASP Collaborative Group (1994) CLASP: a randomised trial of low-dose aspirin for the prevention and treatment of pre-eclampsia among 9364 women. *Lancet.* **343**: 619–26.

CHAPTER 4

Pre-eclampsia and eclampsia

Sandra McDonald

Pre-eclampsia

Pre-eclampsia may be described as an unpredictable and progressive condition with the potential to cause multi-organ dysfunction and failure that can be detrimental to the woman's health and negatively impact on the foetal environment.[1] The incidence of pre-eclampsia in the UK seems to have eluded quantification, but Douglas and Redman[2] indicated that eclampsia complicated one in every 2000 pregnancies. While fatalities associated with pre-eclampsia in the UK are relatively low when compared with other parts of the world, any foetal death causes anguish and a maternal death is an unimaginable tragedy for the family concerned, and is possibly an indicator of failure in the care system.

Midwives at the forefront of maternity care delivery are ideally placed for primary surveillance and early detection of pre-eclampsia. The follow-up activities in which they engage once the condition has been detected will determine the timing of maternal entry into the secondary or tertiary level of care. This can prevent an emergency situation occurring and is thus instrumental to the outcome of any individual pregnancy. Midwives must therefore be especially thorough in the care they provide, and must use knowledge of contemporary research and valid literary evidence to inform their practice and clinical decision-making, ensuring that no action or omission in the exercise of their professional role directly contributes to morbidity or mortality.

While it is not within the remit of this chapter to provide a thorough exposé of the patho-physiology of pre-eclampsia, it is necessary to look at the ways in which the disease process affects the activities of the midwife in the screening process. The initial difficulty lies in definition and the conflicting terminologies used to describe this medical condition which complicates pregnancy. All practitioners will be familiar with what has become the standard description of pre-eclampsia, i.e. 'the occurrence of hypertension, oedema and proteinuria after 20 weeks' gestation in a previously normotensive woman'.[3] However there are uncertainties and dilemmas related to this definition such as, for example, the exact blood pressure measurements that are to be used in defining hypertension, the quantitative value of proteinuria measured and the fact that oedema is a physiologically normal clinical event in the latter part of pregnancy. Further subdivisions are made as to whether the condition should be defined as mild or severe based on the proffered criteria.

The implication of these uncertainties for the practitioner is that the practice of midwifery remains a synergy of art and science. Some women with relatively high blood pressures developed during pregnancy may not seem to have an apparently progressive disease and their babies continue to thrive. Others may present with proteinuria (in which contaminant and infection has been excluded), have pronounced clinical oedema and indications of intrauterine growth restriction of the foetus, but still have normal blood pressure. An even smaller number will show no traditionally acceptable evidence of pre-eclampsia, but present with a non-specific history of feeling unwell and only biochemical investigations reveal the true nature of the disease.

Although it is acknowledged that pre-eclampsia is a very unpredictable disease and may occur in those with no predisposing factors, it may be useful to consider those who have been identified as being at increased risk of developing this condition (see Box 4.1).

Box 4.1: Risk factors for pre-eclampsia[4]

- Primigravida.

- Pre-eclampsia in a previous pregnancy.

- Very young woman or woman over the age of 30 years.

- Second or subsequent pregnancy with a new partner.

- History of pre-eclampsia in mother or sister.

- Women with partners who fathered a previous pre-eclamptic pregnancy.

- Multiple pregnancy.

- History of essential hypertension before pregnancy.

- Hydrop fetalis, hydatidiform mole or polyhydramnios.

- Women with pre-existing medical conditions, e.g. diabetics or renal disease.

Pathophysiology

The aetiology of pre-eclampsia remains unknown, but understanding of the pathogenesis has been advanced in recent years by laboratory work and evidence is becoming increasingly available that the various theories presented have some common features.[5] In a healthy pregnancy uncomplicated by pre-eclampsia, trophoblastic cells invade the maternal uterine arteries at both the decidual and myometrial level resulting in erosion of the muscle layer and enlargement of the lumen.[6] Additionally, there is increased synthesis of prostacyclin,

nitric oxide and thromboxane A_2, which create a change in homeostatic balance and tendency to vasodilatation of the uterine arteries.[7] This alteration in function results in lowered resistance in the arteries, absence of maternal vasomotor control and a massive increase in blood supply to the placenta to meet the demands of the developing foetus.[8] The associated changes account for the transient lowering of maternal blood pressure seen in early pregnancy, which is then compensated for by the physiologic haemodilution.

The probability of a dominant single gene has been suggested as a causative factor in pre-eclampsia and this is thought to affect the level of trophoblastic invasion of the placental bed spiral arteries.[7,9] As a result of arrested trophoblastic invasion adrenergic nerve supplies to the uterine spiral arteries are not disrupted, systemic vascular resistance remains high and placental perfusion is poor. The resultant effect is tissue hypoxia, which is believed to cause liberation of substances that are toxic to endothelial cells; further damage occurs which results in the release of endothelin, a powerful vasoconstrictor.[10] Enhanced contraction of damaged blood vessels facilitates aggregation of platelets at the site of injury.[5] Production of oxygen free radicals, failure of haemodilution, reduced glomerular filtration and poor renal re-absorption all combine to give the presentation seen in pre-eclampsia and are used as the first probable diagnostic signs by the midwife in clinical practice.[10]

Blood pressure

Practitioners are cautioned that any rise in blood pressure occurring after 20 weeks' gestation in a previously normotensive woman should be cause for concern, as this may be the first indicator of a progressive disorder.[5] However, while not underestimating the significance of a rise in blood pressure in combination with other clinical features, it has been suggested that in isolation such a rise may have little effect on the pregnancy, especially in the last trimester.[11]

A diastolic blood pressure recording of 90 mmHg has long been accepted as one sign of pre-eclampsia, but in isolation may not necessarily be unsafe if it plateaus at this level. However a progressive rise is associated with an increase in maternal and neonatal morbidity and mortality.[11] The *Report on Confidential Enquiries into Maternal*

Deaths has included suggested treatment guidelines that define hypertension as 140/90 and severe hypertension as greater than 160/110.[12]

The widespread availability of antenatal care and practice within the above guidelines has given rise to increased surveillance and detection of pre-eclampsia. The results have been timely intervention, improvement in women's care and managed delivery of the baby, all of which have led to a reduction in the number of women seen with severe pre-eclampsia, eclampsia and the accompanying complications involving the liver, lungs and brain.[11,13]

The practising midwife can combine the above information and her knowledge of physiology when screening women for pre-eclampsia. Equally, she needs to be aware of other factors such as any recent physical activity undertaken, the emotions of the woman and the time of day the blood pressure is recorded, as all of these may have an impact upon the accuracy of her observation. The midwife may not have knowledge of the woman's blood pressure before pregnancy at her disposal, because the only recording available as a baseline is usually taken after the early physiological haemodilution, making a later rise of indeterminable significance.

The most recent *Report on Confidential Enquiries into Maternal Deaths* has warned against exclusive reliance on automated blood pressure recording systems.[12] While useful for establishing a trend over several readings, conventional mercury sphygmomanometers remain the instrument of choice in order to prevent underestimation of the blood pressure.

If, in addition to the woman's personal fluctuations, the possibilities of 'white coat syndrome', work stress, less than perfect auditory acuity and a noisy working environment are considered, it can be seen that blood pressure recording is anything but straightforward or simple.[14]

Proteinuria

No dispute seems to exist in the literature as to the importance of proteinuria in the diagnosis of pre-eclampsia, but what is debatable is the amount of protein considered significant. The reagent strips ('dipsticks') commonly used in clinical practice should be considered a guide only to the presence of protein in the urine and not be accepted as an accurate quantification of protein excretion.[15]

When any amount of protein is detected, a clean caught mid-stream sample of urine should be tested to exclude the possibility of contamination. If protein is still detectable, the sample should be sent to the laboratory for exclusion of infection and a 24-hour urine collection should be obtained for protein assessment. It has been suggested that an excess of 0.3 g in a 24-hour collection or an excess of 0.1 g/l of protein in at least two clean samples collected more than six hours apart on separate occasions is an indication of severe fulminating pre-eclampsia.[3]

Practitioners are reminded that the quantity of protein present in urine samples is not indicative of renal damage, but instead is a reflection of capillary leakage and more accurately a projection of the development of generalised oedema. Where protein loss is significant, the possibility of pulmonary and cerebral oedema as complications of pre-eclampsia are considerable.

While the combination of two of the cardinal signs, proteinuria and hypertension, are acceptable as reasonable predictors of worsening pre-eclampsia, it is as well to remember that women with diastolic blood pressures below 90 mmHg or in whom proteinuria was absent have had eclamptic fits.[2,16] The obvious presence of a single finding should prompt investigations for others by measuring known biochemical markers. While the midwife may initiate many of the early biochemical and haematological investigations necessary to obtain a diagnosis, she must remember the scope of her clinical practice. While being eminently able to interpret findings as a measure of the woman's condition, she must always act in accordance with the *Midwives Rules and Code of Practice* and refer the woman to a registered medical practitioner when there are signs of deviation from normal.[17]

Therapy for reducing hypertension

An array of hypotensive treatments have been used to minimise the risk of cerebral damage associated with pre-eclampsia, but it must be borne in mind that these are not cures as they do not arrest the disease progression. A brief description of the mode of action of some of the more popular drugs used in the past to manage pre-eclampsia follows.

Angiotensin converting enzyme (ACE) inhibitors

ACE inhibitors are powerful hypotensive agents that reduce blood pressure by stimulating vasodilation and inhibiting the enzyme necessary for converting angiotensin I to angiotensin II (the latter being a powerful vasoconstrictor). While highly effective for controlling hypertension in non-pregnant individuals they had limited success in pregnancy and are no longer used as one research trial found them to be related to foetal skeletal defects.[18]

Central alpha-II agonist: methyldopa

This is a centrally acting hypotensive drug used in the first line of management in pregnancy. It is an alpha-II agonist acting directly on the brainstem to create vasodilation and lowering of the blood pressure without adverse changes in heart rate, cardiac output, renal perfusion or uteroplacental blood flow.[19] Lowering of the blood pressures is slow, thus where rapid onset of hypotension is desired an alternative drug is preferable.

Alpha and beta sympathetic blocking agents: labetalol, metoprolol and atenolol

This group of peripheral-acting sympatholytic drugs includes alpha, beta and combined alpha + beta sympathetic blocking agents. They act on blood vessels by altering the baroreceptor sympathetic reflex response of nerve to adrenergic vasoconstrictors such as prostaglandins. The resultant effects are maintained vascular relaxation, lowered peripheral resistance and reduced cardiac output, and thus lowering of blood pressure.

Arteriolar dilator: hydralazine

Hydralazine is often reserved for use in cases of very high blood pressure. Given intravenously, it acts directly on the smooth muscles of the arterial wall to bring about vasodilation in ten to 20 minutes with the hypotensive effect lasting six to eight hours. Side effects are headaches, nausea and vomiting (signs which mimic impending eclampsia) and a possible link to thrombocytopenia in the neonate has been reported.

Calcium channel blockers: nifedipine (Adalat®)

This drug belongs to the group of calcium antagonists and has increasingly been used in pre-eclampsia as the second line in hypertensive management where early treatment with methyldopa and sympatholytic agents has failed to keep maternal blood pressure below the danger level. It may be swallowed whole or absorbed sublingually, although some authorities suggest the sublingual route should not be used because mucosal absorption is unpredictable.[20] The effect of the drug is rapid. It works by preventing transfer of calcium ions from extracellular space and inhibits uptake by smooth muscle cells. Vascular muscle response and reflex excitation contractility is reduced and relaxation is achieved, peripheral resistance is lowered and blood vessels dilate, blood pressure falls and the potential for strain on the heart is reduced.[21]

Specific warning is given against the administration of magnesium sulphate where nifedipine has previously been taken and against taking the drug with grapefruit or grapefruit juice, as both these combinations increase the plasma concentration and thus the potency of the drug.[20,22]

Arterial and venous dilator: sodium nitroprusside

This powerful arterial and venous dilator is reserved for use in emergencies. It acts by interfering with intracellular activation of calcium and its effect is immediate but of short duration.[21]

The general consensus of opinion is that hypotensive therapy for managing pre-eclampsia may in some instances when started early in pregnancy prolong the time before hospital admission and commencement of more intensive surveillance and treatment. Drug therapy may therefore prevent the development of very severe hypertension and so avert the development of seizure, and reduce the risks of cerebrovascular accidents, emergency and preterm delivery of the baby, as well as the accompanying perinatal risks.

The choice of which drug is used in practice should probably be related to familiarity as this does instil confidence, a factor essential to the prompt and successful management of the woman's condition. However when scientific evidence indicates that further improvement could be made to this management, it is imperative that practitioners avail themselves of the theoretical knowledge and change practice as necessary.

HELLP syndrome

Serological assessment of the pre-eclamptic woman is an essential component of her care and a rapidly changing profile will warn of deterioration. HELLP syndrome (haemolysis, elevated liver enzymes and low platelets) is a serious complication usually associated with pre-eclampsia and its development is a clear indication for delivery of the foetus.[23] Diagnosis is based on a combination of laboratory findings and clinical signs and symptoms (see Box 4.2), although these may vary significantly.

Box 4.2: HELLP syndrome[23]

Signs and symptoms

- Right upper quadrant pain.

- Epigastric pain.

- Nausea and vomiting.

- Malaise.

- Fatigue.

- Headache.

- Gastro-intestinal bleed.

- Hypertension.

- Proteinuria.

- Reduced urine output.

Laboratory findings

- Haemolysis.

- Anaemia.

- Low platelet count <100 000 mm³.

- Elevated liver enzymes:

  - alanine aminotransferase

  - aspartate aminotransferase

  - gamma glutanyltransferase.

- Elevated levels of bilirubin.

The full blood count is an invaluable screening tool in this process, as evidence of anaemia may indicate excessive breakdown of red cells and can be one of the early features of HELLP. Whether anaemia is due to haemolysis or iron deficiency, it must be borne in mind that its presence will increase the cardiac workload and thus exacerbate hypertension. Alternatively a haemoglobin level which is high for pregnancy may be an indicator of haemoconcentration with reduced intravascular volume and secondary to marked oedema.

The life span of platelets in pre-eclampsia can be reduced by approximately 50% (from nine to five days). Additionally there is an increased level of activation and enhanced adhesion capacity at the site of endothelial cell damage. The combined effect of these changes lead to a continuing fall in platelet count and development of thrombocytopenia, while the multisystem failure can be identified by changes in renal and hepatic function.

Reduced circulatory volume, ischaemia, renal tubular necrosis and reduced renal clearance lead to a rise in the levels of urea, creatinine and serum urate which are indicators of marked maternal and foetal compromise. Infarctions and oedema occurring in the liver will impair its capacity to maintain adequate metabolic activities such as synthesis of clotting factors, while increase in liver size may lead to capsular rupture triggering a combined medical, surgical and obstetric emergency.

Management of HELLP syndrome

Immediate hospitalisation is required to enable more intense monitoring of the maternal and foetal condition with the aim of stabilisation and expediting the birth (see Box 4.3). The time available for measures to be initiated is dictated by the woman's condition, foetal maturity and the clinical facilities available for safe delivery and management of a possible preterm infant. For some women the condition may develop rapidly and before a stage where foetal viability is a possibility, while for others the progression of disease may be more gradual.

Where timing permits, in that the woman's condition does not present an immediate threat, strategies may be implemented to assess foetal well-being and improve survival rates. This may

> **Box 4.3:** Optimal management of HELLP syndrome[24]
>
> - Timely diagnosis.
>
> - Accurate assessment of the severity.
>
> - Control of blood pressure.
>
> - Prevention of seizure.
>
> - Management of fluid and electrolytes balance.
>
> - Assessment of foetal condition.
>
> - Planning and management of delivery.
>
> - Judicious care to manage the potential for haemorrhage.
>
> - Maximum supportive care to enhance the baby's survival.
>
> - Intensive care for the woman post-partum.
>
> - Awareness of the continued risk of multiple organ failure.
>
> - Counselling about future pregnancies.

include biophysical assessment to determine the measure of hypoxaemia and foetal reserve, administration of steroids to accelerate foetal lung maturity in prematurity and continual assessing of foetal well-being by cardiotocography. The woman's condition should also be closely observed for detection of the onset of labour or rapid disease progression, indicated by deterioration in her blood results or increasing severity of physical signs and symptoms.

Fulminating pre-eclampsia

Fulminating pre-eclampsia is a severe medical condition which should be thought of as an emergency. It is essentially a fractional window of opportunity, the duration of which cannot be predicted with any certainty, when timely intervention and appropriate treatment may prevent a seizure. Essentially there are two possible courses of action related to management, either immediate delivery where risk to the woman would be

greater if the pregnancy was continued or prolongation of the pregnancy within a controlled environment once her condition has been stabilised. The latter course will permit administration of corticosteroids to assist foetal lung maturity and benefit the baby which will be born early. While an active search and treat programme is the goal of antenatal care, it offers no guarantee against development of severe pre-eclampsia or eclampsia and it is important that midwifery practitioners know that convulsion may be the first and only indication of an underlying pathological process.[25]

Changes associated with a worsening condition do not necessarily follow a logical, sequential or linear progression, nor are seizures predictable.[26] Some women may have very severe presentation of pre-eclampsia where the practitioner expects the condition to culminate in convulsion, yet this does not happen. Therefore it is imperative that midwives remain watchful for new developments or subtle changes discernible through close physical observation and changes in levels of biochemical tests, but not let observation or test results diminish attentiveness or create a false sense of security.

Blood pressure

The importance of blood pressure measurement has been introduced above, but in severe pre-eclampsia observations are made and recorded at intervals of between five and fifteen minutes and are closely balanced by administration of medication in accordance with prescribed instructions. The purpose of this is to ensure an appropriate response that is finely balanced to avert seizure, yet protect against the occurrence of sudden devastating hypotension that can be detrimental to the woman's cerebral function and foetal well-being.

Renal function

In pregnancy urea and creatinine clearance is high, but blood levels at the upper end of the range may be suggestive of impaired renal clearance, while a marked rise in creatinine is indicative of severe renal impairment.

A rise in serum uric acid production is secondary to tissue ischaemia and increasing levels may be reflective of impaired renal clearance, renal medullary ischaemia and tubular damage.[15] These findings may be the only clinical indicators of the seriousness of pre-eclampsia. The importance of this information is that a rise in serum uric acid can be detected before protein-uria becomes evident. Leakage of albumin through the kidneys is a positive indication of glomerular endothelial damage, the conse-quences of which are lowering of serum albumin levels and leakage of fluid into the extra cellular space.

Low levels of serum albumin will result in excessive loss of intravascular volume, impact on the cardiovascular system and be evident as oedema. This is indicated as a rise in haematocrit, polycythaemia, reducing renal perfusion, impaired renal tubular function and poor reabsorption of protein, causing further leakage of fluid into the extra cellular space and resulting in reduced urinary output – a vicious cycle is in motion. The woman should be catheterised, and the urine measured hourly (output should be 0.5 ml/kg/hr and should not fall below 30 ml/hr) and tested for the quantity of protein.

Liver function

Raised levels of liver enzymes such as alanine aminotransferase, aspartate aminotransferase and bilirubin, in combination with placental alkaline phosphatase, are indicators of a significant level of liver cell damage and the development of HELLP syndrome.[27]

Development of epigastric or left upper quadrant pain is indicative of liver involvement. Damage to the endothelial lining of blood vessels in the liver results in leakage of plasma and causes an increase in size and overstretching of the fibrous capsule. In addition, blood vessels may rupture and haematoma may form in the sub-capsular region, increasing the pressure on the liver peritoneum with referred pain.

While the damage to the liver caused by HELLP syndrome resolves spontaneously in the postpartum period, there is a need for the midwife to be aware of differential causes of abdominal pain. For example, acute fatty liver disease is a dangerous condition of unknown origin that can complicate pre-eclampsia and because presentation is similar to pre-eclampsia, with symptoms of headache, abdominal pain, vomiting and reduced urinary output, it is difficult to identify.

Serology

A full blood count is a valuable assessment in pre-eclampsia as much information can be gained. Normal pregnancy results in physiological haemodilution and lower levels of erythrocytes in a specified volume of blood, although their life span is not affected. In pre-eclampsia the reduction in intravascular volume causes a rise in haematocrit and polycythaemia, while erythrocytes are damaged by their forced passage and friction with the damaged endothelial lining of blood vessels. Repeated damage significantly reduces the life expectancy of erythrocytes leading to increased haemolysis and anaemia.

Mild thrombocytopenia, the cause of which is unknown, has long been identified as an uncom-plicated finding in normal pregnancy, but when present in pre-eclampsia the platelet levels should be closely and regularly monitored. Acute presentation (indicated by a fall of between 20–30% from the baseline measurement in early pregnancy) is associated with severe pre-eclampsia and HELLP syndrome. It is thought to be related to a shorter life span of the platelets and aggregation at the site of endothelial vascular damage, secondary to the hypertensive state.

Walker[15] suggests that a falling platelet count could be used as a guide to the timing of delivery, as it is associated with a worsening of the maternal and foetal condition. Adhesion of platelets to damaged endothelial blood vessel walls narrows the lumen, reduces end organ perfusion, exacer-bates tissue damage through anoxia and pre-disposes the woman to development of eclampsia, placental abruption and possible foetal demise.[15]

Care of the woman with fulminating pre-eclampsia

Women admitted with fulminating or severe pre-eclampsia must be closely monitored (see Box 4.4) and medicated. One-to-one care, with drugs and equipment for managing an eclamptic fit, monitoring the foetal condition and supporting adequate ventilation and oxygen therapy, is essential. A multidisciplinary approach involving obstetrician and anaesthetist at consultant level, haematologist, paediatrician and appropriately experienced midwife should be involved in the

Box 4.4: Signs and symptoms of fulminating eclampsia[27,28]

- Continuing rise in blood pressure.

- Increasing proteinuria.

- Oliguria.

- Development of epigastric pain.

- Nausea and vomiting.

- Severe headache.

- Visual field disturbance (floaters or diplopia).

- Bleeding tendency.

- Jaundice.

- Deep tendon reflex.

- Clonus.

planning and provision of care, and the neonatal intensive care unit should be put on stand-by.

Management of the woman's condition necessitates two aims being pursued simultaneously, namely lowering of the blood pressure and intensive observation of maternal and foetal condition. The first objective requires initiation of therapy to reduce the blood pressure to a level where the potential for seizure is reduced, thereby protecting the woman's cerebrovascular circulation and preventing a stroke.[28] A level of blood pressure around 140/90 mmHg is thought to be a safe compromise as further reductions may well impair placental perfusion and affect foetal well-being.[27] The second objective involves intense monitoring of maternal and foetal condition for early detection of deterioration (impending seizure, organ failure, and pulmonary oedema), the onset of labour and/or evidence of foetal compromise.

The midwife must record vital signs at least every 15 minutes with particular attention being paid to blood pressure and level of consciousness. Medication being used for control of blood pressure should be administered as prescribed, while intake and output levels and central venous pressure (CVP) readings should be measured and recorded. The urine should be tested frequently and the amount of protein quantified. Continuous

monitoring of the foetal heart rate pattern is essential.

Nil-by-mouth is usual and intravenous access is essential. Hartmann's solution may be used with strict control of the rate of infusion (usually approximately 50 ml/hr or 1000 ml/24 hr), to reduce the risk of cardiac failure and pulmonary oedema. As a very fine balance between intake and output is required, this is best achieved by monitoring of the CVP which should be maintained at around 4–6 mmHg.[29] Clinical biochemical features of full blood count, electrolytes, uric acid, liver enzymes, fibrinogen, platelets, clotting studies and blood urea nitrogen (BUN) should be assessed every four hours or daily as the woman's condition dictates.

If the woman's condition stabilises sufficiently to enable labour to be induced, an epidural analgesia is often selected where the clotting studies are satisfactory. This method of pain relief offers the additional benefits of lowering blood pressure, elimination of painful stimuli that may trigger convulsion and avoids the possibility of anaesthetic complications which may accompany general anaesthesia and exacerbate pulmonary oedema.

There is a 1:200 risk of eclampsia where the woman has had pre-eclampsia, if any difficulty is encountered in achieving control of the blood pressure, or there are indications of HELLP syndrome, fulminating pre-eclampsia or foetal distress. Therefore such measures as are necessary to hasten foetal lung maturity must be initiated and delivery must be expedited.[15] Effective measures are needed to prevent convulsion, major organ failure, foetal demise, and reduce the severity of postpartum exacerbation and long term morbidity. However, once a convulsion has occurred the continuation of the pregnancy cannot be justified.

Eclampsia

Eclampsia is the occurrence of convulsions that are associated with the signs and symptoms of pre-eclampsia.[2] It is a Greek word meaning lightning and often strikes with the same random ferocity and has similarly devastating effects. The seizure that is the key feature of eclampsia is thought to be due to intense vasospasm of the cerebral arteries, oedema secondary to ischaemic damage of vascular endothelium and intravascular clot formation.[30]

Box 4.5: Midwifery care of the woman with fulminating pre-eclampsia

- Monitor blood pressure.

- Monitor and record urinary output and level of proteinuria.

- Administer drugs and titrate according to blood pressure response.

- Monitor foetal condition and assess for onset of labour.

- Maintain a quiet calm atmosphere.

- Monitor blood results for detection of changes reflecting deterioration.

- Assess for symptoms of worsening condition.

- Provide psychological care for the woman and her family.

- Any significant changes in the woman's condition must be notified to the obstetrician and/or anaesthetist.

An eclamptic fit usually includes three defined phases.

1 Prodromal, in which the imminent fit is heralded by possible report of visual disturbances, muscular twitching, facial congestion, foaming at the mouth and/or deepening loss of consciousness.

2 Tonoclonic, where initially generalised muscular contractions are present and respiration is absent. This is followed by repeated strong jerky irregular muscular activity.

3 Abatement, which occurs within 1–1½ minutes of onset during which time respiration is re-established and there is gradual return to consciousness, but perhaps with a confused and agitated state.

It is futile to attempt any action within the short interval of the tonoclonic phase apart from protecting the woman from injury. However subsequent care should be aimed at damage limitation by placing the woman in the recovery position once the seizure has passed. Suction should be used to clear secretions from the mouth and nasal passage to maintain a clear airway and oxygen should be administered. These immediate measures help to boost the maternal oxygen saturation and improve delivery to the foetus which would have been deprived of oxygen during the tonoclonic phase of the seizure. Further urgent measures are now imperative to

prevent the recurrence of further seizure and optimise maternal and foetal well-being (*see* Box 4.6).

Various therapies combining hypotensive agents and anticonvulsants have been used in recent times to manage pre-eclampsia and eclampsia, but without any consensus on efficacy. Recent research studies carried out in the USA and UK comparing treatments of eclampsia concluded that magnesium sulphate was effective both as an anticonvulsant and hypotensive agent.[31,32,33,34] However although magnesium sulphate is best for preventing recurrence of fits, it is not known if it is the best prophylactic.[35]

Suggested treatment regime using magnesium sulphate

Suggested loading and maintenance doses are given in Table 4.1. As magnesium sulphate is a powerful depressant of neuromuscular transmission, extreme care must be taken to avoid sudden hypotension. Additionally, as this drug is excreted via the kidneys, existing damage and impaired clearance could result in toxic levels being quickly reached. A maximum blood magnesium level of 4 mmol/l is therapeutic, but around 7 mmol/l is associated with respiratory distress, while levels of around 12 mmol/l can trigger cardiac arrest. The frequency with which serum magnesium levels are measured will depend on

Box 4.6: Immediate care of the eclamptic woman

- Summon assistance (anaesthetist and obstetrician).
- Protect from injury during the tono-clonic phase.
- Maintain airway (clear by suctioning if necessary).
- Provide supplementary oxygenation.
- Place woman in the left lateral (recovery) position.
- Obtain intravenous access and monitor fluid balance.
- Treat the convulsion.
- Possibly sedate to prevent hyper-stimulation.
- Monitor vital signs.
- Assess foetal well-being (risk of foetal distress from hypoxia or abruption).
- Achieve stability of maternal condition.
- Plan mode of delivery.
- Execute plan without further delay.

Box 4.7: Signs and symptoms of magnesium sulphate toxicity

- Loss of tendon reflexes.
- Double vision.
- Depressed respiration.
- Slurred speech.
- Flushing.
- Weakness.
- Reduced urinary output <0.5 ml/kg/hr.
- Drowsiness.

may be many questions the woman wishes to have answered. The skills of the midwife as communicator will be essential in providing information that is timely, appropriate, accurate and as comprehensive as possible to assist with the process of adjustment to what has been a life-threatening event.

References

1 Munro PT (2000) Management of eclampsia in the accident and emergency department. *J Accid Emerg Med.* **17**: 7–11.
2 Douglas KA and Redman CWG (1994) Eclampsia in the UK. *BMJ.* **309**: 1395–8.
3 Witlin AG and Sibai BM (1997) Hypertension in pregnancy: current concepts of pre-eclampsia. *Ann Rev Med.* **48**: 115–27.
4 Dekker GA (1999) Risk factors for pre-eclampsia. *Clin Obstet and Gynecol.* **42** (3): 422–35.
5 Zhang J, Zeisler J, Hatch MC and Berkowits G (1997) Epidemiology of pregnancy induced hypertension. *Epidemiol Rev.* **19** (2): 218–32.

urinary output as an indicator of renal function and the presence of positive screening characteristics are indicative of approaching toxicity levels (*see* Box 4.7).

Once the woman's condition has stabilised and the baby has been delivered, the aggressive approach to management needs to be maintained as the risk of eclamptic fits occurring during the first 24 hours of the postpartum period remains. In addition to the physical care the woman requires, there is the need for psychological support as there

Table 4.1: Suggested doses of magnesium sulphate

	Dose
Loading dose	Intravenous: 4 g in 20% solution over 5–15 min followed by Slow infusion: 5 g in 500 ml normal saline at a rate of 1 g/hr
Maintenance dose	Continue the slow infusion as above for at least 24 hours after last convulsion or delivery.

6 Hytten F and Chamberlain G (1980) *Clinical Physiology in Obstetrics*. Blackwell Scientific, Oxford.

7 Meekins JW, Pijnenborg R, Hanssen M et al. (1994) A study of placental bed spiral arteries and trophoblast invasion in normal and severe pre-eclamptic pregnancies. *Br J Obstet Gynaecol.* **101**: 669–74.

8 Dekker GA and Sibai BM (1998) Etiology and pathogenesis of pre-eclampsia: current concepts. *Am J Obstet Gynecol.* **179** (5): 1359–79.

9 Liston WA and Kilpatrick DG (1991) Is genetic susceptibility to pre-eclampsia conferred by homozygosity for the same single recessive gene in mother and fetus? *Br J Obstet Gynaecol.* **98**: 1079–86.

10 Halliwell B (1994) Free radicals, antioxidants and human disease: curiosity, cause or consequence? *Lancet.* **344**: 721–4.

11 Duley L and Henderson-Smart DJ (2000) Drugs for rapid treatment of very high blood pressure in pregnancy. In: *The Cochrane Library* (Issue 4). Update Software, Oxford.

12 Lewis G (ed) (2001) *Why Mothers Die 1997–1999: the fifth report of the confidential enquiries into maternal deaths in the United Kingdom*. RCOG Press, London.

13 Department of Health (1998) *Why Mothers Die: report on confidential enquiries into maternal deaths in the United Kingdom 1994–1996*. The Stationery Office, London.

14 Foster C (1995) Professional development: blood pressure; knowledge for practice; the role of the nurse; revision notes. *Nurs Times.* **91**: 1–14.

15 Walker JJ (2000) Severe pre-eclampsia and eclampsia. *Baillières Clin Obstet Gynaecol.* **14** (1): 57–71.

16 Sibai BM (1990) Eclampsia VI. Maternal-perinatal outcome in 254 consecutive cases. *Am J Obstet Gynecol.* **163**: 1049–55.

17 United Kingdom Central Council for Nursing, Midwifery and Health Visiting (1998) *Midwives Rules and Code of Practice*. UKCC, London.

18 Hanssens M, Keirse MJNC, Vankelecom F and Assche FA (1991) Fetal and neonatal effects of treatment with ACE inhibitors in pregnancy. *Obstet Gynecol.* **78**: 128.

19 Usta IM and Sibai BM (1995) Emergency management of puerperal eclampsia: intrapartum and postpartum obstetric emergencies. *Obstet Gynecol Clin N Am.* **22**: 315–35.

20 Churchill D and Beevers DG (1999) Treatment of hypertensive disorders of pregnancy. In: D Churchill and DG Beevers (eds) *Hypertension in Pregnancy*. BMJ Books, London.

21 Witlin AG and Sibai BM (1997) Hypertension in pregnancy: current concepts of pre-eclampsia. *Ann Rev Med.* **48**: 115–27.

22 Pfizer (2000) *Istin: summary of product characteristics*. Pfizer, Sandwich.

23 Egerman RS and Sibai BM (1999) HELLP syndrome. *Clin Obstet Gynecol.* **42** (2): 381–8.

24 Magann EF and Martin JN (1999) Twelve steps to optimal management of HELLP Syndrome. *Clin Obstet and Gynecol.* **42** (3): 532–50.

25 Witling AG and Sibai BM (1998) Magnesium sulphate therapy in pre-eclampsia and eclampsia. *Obstet Gynecol.* **92**: 883–9.

26 Kats VL, Farmer R and Kuller JA (2000) Pre-eclampsia into eclampsia: towards a new paradigm. *Am J Obstet Gynecol.* **182** (6): 1389–96.

27 Chamberlain G and Steer P (1999) ABC of labour care: labour in special circumstances. *BMJ.* **318** (7191): 1124–7.

28 Symonds EM (1995) Hypertension in Pregnancy. *Arch Dis Childhood* (Fetal and Neonatal Edition). **72** (2): 77–83.

29 Moodley J, Jjuuko G and Rout C (2001) Epidural compared with general anaesthetic for caesarean section delivery in conscious women with eclampsia. *Br J Obstet and Gynaecol.* **108**: 378–82.

30 Felz MW, Barnes DB and Figuero RM (2000) Late postpartum eclampsia 16 days after delivery: case report with clinical, radiologic and patho-physiologic correlation. *J Am Board Fam Pract.* **13** (1): 39–46.

31 Crowther C (1990) Magnesium sulphate versus diazepam in management of eclampsia: a randomized controlled trial. *Br J Obstet Gynaecol.* **97**: 110–17.

32 Dommisse J (1990) Phenytoin sodium and magnesium sulphate in management of eclampsia. *Br J Obstet Gynaecol.* **97**: 104–9.

33 Appleton MP, Kuchl TJ, Raebel MA, Adams HR, Knight AB and Gold WR (1991) Magnesium sulphate versus phenytoin for seizure prophylaxis in pregnancy-induced hypertension. *Am J Obstet Gynecol.* **165**: 907–13.

34 Belfort MA and Moise KJ (1992) Effect of magnesium sulphate on maternal brain blood flow in pre-eclampsia: a randomized, placebo controlled study. *Am J Obstet Gynecol.* **167**: 661–6.

35 Duley L (1996) Magnesium sulphate regimens for women with eclampsia: messages from the collaborative eclampsia trial. *Br J Obstet Gynaecol.* **103**: 103–5.

CHAPTER 5

Antepartum haemorrhage

Hazel Sundle

Introduction

Antepartum haemorrhage occurs in approximately 2–3% of all pregnancies and can be defined as bleeding from the genital tract after 24 weeks' gestation and before the birth of the baby. If the woman is in labour, similar bleeding is called intrapartum haemorrhage (*see* Chapter 10). The types of haemorrhage can be described as:

- accidental: as in placental abruption
- incidental: from local lesions in the genital tract
- inevitable: as in placenta praevia.

Any bleeding in pregnancy can be potentially dangerous if it leads to foetal or maternal compromise. Third trimester bleeding is still a main cause of perinatal morbidity and mortality. The most common causes of dangerous bleeding in the latter part of pregnancy are placental abruption (abruptio placentae), and placenta praevia. Approximately just over half of the women who present with an antepartum haemorrhage are found to have one of these two conditions. There is often no firm diagnosis made for the other half, whose bleeding is said to be unclassified or bleeding of unknown origin.[1]

It is recommended that women presenting with any vaginal bleeding should be followed up carefully antenatally to monitor the bleeding and foetal well-being, as such bleeding is associated with a high perinatal mortality rate.[2] According to the most recent *Report on Confidential Enquiries into Maternal Deaths* there were three deaths due to placental abruption and three to placenta praevia from 1997–99.[3]

Risk or predisposing factors

The predisposing factors of placental abruption and placenta praevia are shown in Table 5.1 and discussed below.

Threatened miscarriage

Obed and Adewole[4] studied the antenatal and labour records of 374 pregnant women who had prior diagnosis of threatened miscarriage, to look for the incidence of placental abruption and placenta praevia. These were compared with the records of 500 women without a history of threatened miscarriage. They found that first trimester threatened miscarriage was associated with about two and a half times the risk of placental abruption and placenta praevia compared with that of the general obstetric population. They suggest that women with such a history should be followed closely throughout their pregnancy, especially ensuring placental localisation.

Previous caesarean section

There is evidence from several sources to suggest that women who have had a previous caesarean section are more at risk of developing placenta praevia.[5,6,7,8]

History of miscarriage and induced abortion

Ananth et al.[6] wanted to quantify the risk of placenta praevia based on the number of previous caesarean deliveries and a history of miscarriage and induced abortion from the available epidemiological evidence. They found a strong association between having a previous caesarean delivery, spontaneous or induced abortion and the subsequent development of placenta praevia. They also found that the risk increased with the number of previous caesareans and suggested that these women must be regarded as high risk for developing placenta praevia.

High parity and older age

Similarly, many sources agree that women who have had three or more previous babies are at higher risk of developing placenta praevia.[5,7,9] In addition older women of more than 35 years are widely recognised as being more at risk of developing both abruption and placenta praevia.[9]

Maternal cocaine use

Macones et al.[5] wanted to determine whether maternal cocaine use was a risk factor for placenta praevia. They compared cases of placenta praevia with a random sample of women without placenta praevia. They obtained data regarding cocaine use, along with other potential risk factors, from antenatal records. Their results suggested that along with other predisposing factors such as previous caesarean section, elective abortion and high parity, maternal cocaine use was an independent risk factor.

Smoking

Andres[10] reported that smoking was recognised as having an adverse effect on pregnancy outcome as early as the mid 1950s. He reviewed the published literature written about women who smoked in pregnancy and found that the risk of placental abruption and/or placenta praevia was increased in this group. The risk increased with the number of cigarettes smoked (10 a day or over), and the number of years over which they had smoked (6 years or more). Those women who gave up smoking during their pregnancy were shown to be at no greater risk of developing placental abruption than those who didn't smoke.

Hypertensive disorders

It is widely recognised that hypertensive disorders in pregnancy can predispose to placental abruption.[11,12] Ananth et al.[12] reviewed the literature to evaluate the joint influences of smoking and hypertensive disorders (chronic hypertension and pre-eclampsia) on the subsequent development of abruption. They found an increased risk of placental abruption in relation to both smoking and hypertensive disorders during pregnancy. Severe pre-eclampsia and chronic hypertension with superimposed pre-eclampsia have a strong association with placental abruption.[11]

Multiple pregnancy

Another risk factor for both placenta praevia and abruption is multiple pregnancy. Because there is usually a greater surface area of placental tissue with multiple pregnancies, there is more likelihood of it encroaching on the lower segment. Abruption could result after sudden decompression of the uterine cavity, for example after spontaneous rupture of membranes of the first twin, delivery of the first twin or in cases of polyhydramnios.

Domestic violence

Unfortunately, domestic violence is common against women, although it is very difficult to quantify. Pregnancy seems to be viewed by violent men as a trigger for further abuse.[13,14,15,16] Violent attacks during pregnancy seem to be focused on the abdomen, breasts and genitals.[13] It is thought that this may be because the pregnancy stimulates feelings of jealousy towards the foetus in the male partner, because it represents the transition to becoming a family or because the frequency of sexual intercourse is reduced. Violence is repeatedly shown to be a cause of maternal and perinatal morbidity with an increased risk of placental abruption.[13,14,16] Psychological effects on the pregnant woman subjected to domestic violence may lead her to indulge in drug taking, including smoking and alcohol. Smoking and cocaine use have been shown above to increase the risk of abruption and placenta praevia.

Placental abruption

Placental abruption occurs in about 1:150 deliveries.[17] It can be defined as the complete or partial separation of a normally implanted placenta occurring after 24 weeks' gestation, prior to delivery, usually accompanied by abdominal pain and uterine bleeding, and often confirmed after delivery by evidence of retroplacental bleeding or clot.

The perinatal mortality rate with confirmed abruption is high, often over 300 for every 1000 diagnosed, with more than half the perinatal losses due to foetal death before the mother arrives in hospital.[18]

The haemorrhage can be classified (*see* Figure 5.1) as:

* revealed: the bleeding usually passes between the membranes and the uterus to escape through the cervix and appear *per vaginum*

* *concealed*: the blood remains trapped between the placenta and the uterus

* *mixed*: both of the above occur.

Depending on the degree of separation of the placenta and therefore the condition of the mother and foetus, the severity of the abruption can be described as mild, moderate or severe.

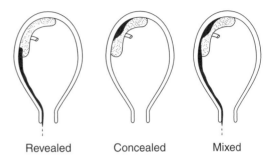

Revealed   Concealed   Mixed

Figure 5.1 Placental abruption

Pathophysiology

Placental separation is triggered by bleeding into the decidua basalis (lining of the uterus) with haematoma formation. The blood clot weighs down and adheres to the maternal surface of the placenta. As the placenta separates, bleeding may track down between the membranes and the uterus and appear externally. This is a revealed haemorrhage. In a concealed haemorrhage, the bleeding is more centrally located, may be retained behind the placenta and can infiltrate into the myometrium (muscle layer of the uterus) causing pain, uterine tenderness and irritability. If this blood infiltration is significant, it is known as a Couvelaire uterus or uterine apoplexy. A haemorrhage of this severity can lead to foetal and/or maternal death, maternal coagulation defects,

Table 5.1: Predisposing factors

Factor	Placental abruption	Placenta praevia
History of first trimester threatened miscarriage	✔	✔
Previous caesarean section	✗	✔
History of spontaneous miscarriage or induced abortion	✗	✔
Parity ≥3	✔	✔
Maternal cocaine use	✔	✔
Smoking	✔	✔
Hypertension	✔	✗
Maternal age	✔	✔
Multiple pregnancy	✔	✔
Domestic violence	✔	✗

renal failure and, rarely, Sheehan's syndrome. A mixed haemorrhage may have some revealed and some concealed bleeding.

Signs and symptoms

Bleeding

As already described, the amount of blood seen when a woman presents with a placental abruption is not associated with the severity of the abruption. The blood may be red if it is fresh loss, but there may be brown blood if it has been retained *in utero* for any length of time.

Shock

The woman's skin may be pale and clammy and her vital signs may suggest hypovolaemic shock (*see* Chapter 2 for further discussion).

Abdominal pain

This can be either moderate or severe, intermittent or continuous. Backache may be present if the placenta is posterior.

Abdominal examination

In a concealed haemorrhage, there may be an increase in abdominal girth and the uterus may be firm or 'board-like' (Couvelaire) on palpation. The abdomen may be tender to touch.

Evidence of foetal distress

The woman may report a history of reduced or excessive foetal movements. The foetal heart may show signs of distress or be absent.

Anxiety

Any deviation from the norm in the progression of pregnancy can cause anxiety in women.

The abruption may be associated with hypertensive disorders or trauma such as a road traffic accident, attempted external cephalic version or abuse.

Placenta praevia

Placenta praevia is where the placenta is partially or wholly implanted in the lower uterine segment on either the anterior or posterior wall. It occurs in about 0.5% of all pregnancies. In grand multiparity the incidence can be as high as 2%.[19] The perinatal mortality rate is now 50–60 in every 1000.[18]

Classification divides placenta praevia into four types (*see* Figure 5.2):

- Type I (lateral or low-lying): the placenta encroaches on the lower uterine segment but does not extend as far as the cervical os
- Type II (marginal): the edge of the placenta extends to the internal cervical os but does not cover it

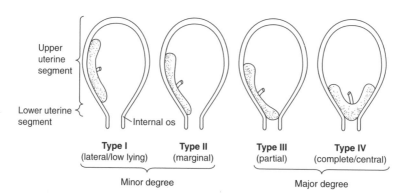

Figure 5.2 Placenta praevia

- Type III (partial): the placenta partially covers the internal os
- Type IV (complete or central): the placenta completely covers the internal os.

Approximately half of all placenta praevia are of minor degree (types I and II), and half are major (types III and IV).[17] About 80% of women with placenta praevia bleed before the onset of labour. Generally, those of major degree bleed earlier in the pregnancy and more heavily than those of minor degree. Lam et al.[20] studied the maternal and neonatal outcomes of 159 women with a diagnosed placenta praevia who bled in their pregnancy compared to 93 who did not. They found that the neonatal outcome was worse in those women who had bled, with more respiratory distress, low Apgar scores and admissions to neonatal unit (accounted for mainly by the higher incidence of prematurity). The same women were also more likely to have had antenatal steroids, tocolytic agents and/or emergency caesarean section delivery.

It is commonplace in the UK for pregnant women to have a routine ultrasound scan at 18–20 weeks' gestation. About 5–6% of all placentae will appear low at this gestation as the lower uterine segment is not yet formed. In these cases, women will be recommended to have a repeat scan at approximately 32 weeks' gestation and should be advised what to do if bleeding occurs before this. Only a minority of the women rescanned will be diagnosed with placenta praevia. Their subsequent management will be decided depending on their individual condition. That means that with placental migration as a result of anatomical changes in the lower segment, 90% of women diagnosed with a low-lying placenta at 20 weeks' gestation will have a normally-sited placenta later in pregnancy.[21]

Signs and symptoms

With placenta praevia, the edge may separate from the uterine wall and cause bleeding which is always visible.

Bleeding

Fresh red loss which is apparently unprovoked. Pain is not a feature because the low-lying placenta allows the blood to escape, thus avoiding the formation of a retroplacental clot. Bleeding could possibly be initiated by coitus.

Shock

This would correspond to the amount of blood loss.

Abdominal palpation

There is often malpresentation and/or unstable lie because the placenta occupies the space in the pelvis where the baby's head usually lies. Breech is particularly common. In any presentation, the presenting part may remain high.

Evidence of foetal distress

The foetal heart is usually normal. Foetal tachycardia may be present and reflect maternal tachycardia. Foetal hypoxia may be present with severe haemorrhage.

Uterus

The uterus is usually soft and non-tender.

Anxiety

Any deviation from the norm in the progression of pregnancy can cause anxiety in women.

Immediate treatment

It is always important to remember that every woman who is experiencing an antepartum haemorrhage is different and should be treated sensitively and individually.

A calm attitude and continual explanation of procedures is paramount in order to instil trust and confidence in the woman and her family. Medical aid should be summoned immediately. *See* Box 5.1 for a list of personnel who may be involved. Obviously, the immediate treatment given will depend on the severity of the haemorrhage and therefore the condition of the mother and foetus. Priority should always be given to resuscitating and stabilising the woman before delivering the baby. The midwife should remember that any bleeding can be serious and the condition of the mother and foetus can deteriorate

Box 5.1: Essential team members for controlling a moderate or severe haemorrhage

- Midwife.

- Labour ward coordinator.

- On-call specialist registrar and senior house officer.

- Consultant obstetrician.

- Blood transfusion service.

- Anaesthetist.

- Haematologist.

- Paediatrician.

- Neonatal unit nursing staff.

- Porters.

- Any other staff to give assistance but not get in the way!

rapidly. If the mother is in pain a narcotic drug may be given.

Initial observation includes assessment for shock by looking for clammy skin, pallor, air hunger and indications from the woman's vital signs. If the woman has a placental abruption with associated hypertension, her blood pressure may not be abnormally low, thus masking the clinical signs of shock.

If the midwife is attending the woman at home, her priority is to transfer her to the nearest consultant-led obstetric unit, ideally with appropriate neonatal facilities. Transfer should be done via the emergency obstetric team or by ambulance in accordance with local policies and procedures. An intravenous infusion should be sited to initiate fluid replacement. The mother should be positioned so as to avoid supine hypotension as this could exacerbate her state of shock and further compromise the foetus.

Neither a digital vaginal nor a rectal examination should be performed as this could aggravate the bleeding. A speculum examination may be carried out to exclude cervical or vaginal lesions as a cause for the bleeding, although this procedure may be considered an unnecessary

procedure by some obstetricians and midwives. Chilaka et al.[22] carried out a study at a UK teaching hospital to determine whether an admission speculum was a necessary routine procedure for all women presenting with antepartum haemorrhage. They found that the complications of pregnancy, timing of delivery and subsequent management were not influenced by the findings from speculum examination. They suggested that this procedure may not be justifiable for all women presenting with antepartum haemorrhage.

Accurate and thorough history-taking will give the team information on the amount of blood loss, any associated pain, trauma, recent sexual intercourse or any previous episodes of bleeding. This will help in trying to determine the cause of the bleeding. The woman may have had a recent scan indicating placental location. She may have had previous hospital admissions with bleeding or hypertension.

Palpation will give an indication of the size of the baby and help to determine the cause of haemorrhage according to whether or not the abdomen is tender, soft or 'board-like'. A history of repeated small bleeds during the pregnancy may have resulted in placental insufficiency which can lead to associated intrauterine growth restriction.

The foetal condition is assessed by initial auscultation, then cardiotocography and a description of the nature of recent foetal movements from the mother.

The following blood tests needed are: full blood count, group and cross match/save, clotting and in cases of hypertension, biochemistry screen (*see* Chapter 4 for details of the pre-eclampsia blood tests). If the mother is rhesus negative, a Kleihauer test should also be done. Intravenous therapy will be administered as necessary to maintain blood pressure and circulating volume.

A scan is necessary in most cases to determine the location of the placenta. Even if this has been done previously in pregnancy, it should be repeated as there have been cases reported where routine pregnancy ultrasound has not been accurate in placental localisation.[23] If the placenta is found to be normally sited, any separation may be seen on ultrasound although this is not always the case.[21]

See Chapter 10 and Box 10.4 for a description of the preparation necessary if an emergency caesarean section is planned.

Further treatment

Placental abruption

After a mild haemorrhage, the condition of the mother and foetus are not normally compromised. The blood loss will probably all be revealed.

If the gestation of the baby is no more than 34 weeks, corticosteroids can be administered to accelerate foetal lung maturity.[24] The woman should be introduced to the neonatal unit staff and a visit to the unit organised. If she is rhesus negative, she should be offered an intramuscular injection of anti-D immunoglobulin with full explanation of its effects. The woman may be allowed home after a few days of observation provided there has been no further bleeding, and frequent monitoring indicates that the foetal heart is normal. The placental site will have been determined by ultrasound scan.

If further bleeding occurs and the gestation is 37 weeks or over then labour may be induced. If this coincides with any signs of foetal distress, delivery by caesarean section may be necessary.

A moderate haemorrhage is where up to one litre of blood has been lost and about one quarter of the placenta separated. The blood loss may be partially concealed and partially revealed – a mixed haemorrhage. The condition of the mother is compromised with shock, abdominal pain and guarding. Regular observation of these signs, as well as accurate measurements of pulse, blood pressure and fluid balance should be made. Analgesia may be required for the mother.

The foetus may have already died or be hypoxic. If it is in good condition or has died, vaginal delivery should be attempted unless there is a contraindication such as transverse lie or malpresentation. The contractions should help to control the bleeding. Enkin et al.[2] suggest that inducing labour, using oxytocin if necessary and continuously monitoring foetal heart rate may result in a 50% reduction of the risk of caesarean section with no significant risk of perinatal mortality.

If the baby is alive but showing signs of distress, caesarean section is the most appropriate mode of delivery once the mother's condition has been stabilised. To treat shock, it is necessary to replace blood loss with appropriate plasma expanders and whole blood so that the baby can be delivered as soon as possible.

With a severe haemorrhage, two or more litres of blood will have been lost and more than half of the placenta separated. It is highly likely that the foetus will be dead. The mother will be shocked, in extreme pain and most of the blood will be concealed behind the placenta. The mother will need a central venous pressure line to monitor fluid, an in-dwelling urinary catheter and analgesia. Although the treatment is the same as for a moderate haemorrhage, the mother is more at risk of coagulation defects, renal failure and pituitary failure. Efficient team work and good communication between the labour ward and blood transfusion laboratories are essential.

Placenta praevia

Management decisions for women with placenta praevia are based on clinical and ultrasound findings. Sunna and Ziadeh[25] carried out a randomised prospective study to evaluate the use of transvaginal (TVS) and transabdominal (TAS) ultrasound in the diagnosis of placenta praevia and its effect on the length of stay in hospital. They suggest that TVS is a safe and more accurate method of scanning than TAS and can reduce the length of hospital stay. The Royal College of Obstetricians and Gynaecologists (RCOG)[26] advocates this method of scanning in their paper on diagnosis and management of placenta praevia.

The RCOG[26] say that if the placenta encroaches within 2 cm of the internal os, then delivery should be by caesarean section. They also specify that the choice of anaesthetic technique must be made by the anaesthetist conducting the procedure. The first bleed suffered by women with placenta praevia does not normally compromise the mother or foetus and is sometimes referred to as a 'warning bleed'. Severe bleeding usually occurs after the 34th week of pregnancy and about 50% of women with placenta praevia deliver at less than 35 weeks.[17]

Induction of labour may be appropriate once the foetus has reached an adequate gestation and the placenta has been classified as low-lying (type I) or marginal (type II). However, an artificial rupture of membranes must only be performed in controlled conditions, i.e. in the operating theatre with blood available in case of haemorrhage. The foetal head should be below the placental edge and amniotomy attempted by a senior obstetrician. If any placental tissue can be felt then the procedure should be abandoned and an emergency caesarean section performed.

Expectant or conservative management is appropriate with slight to moderate bleeding. The object is to minimise the problems of prematurity which are possible when a baby is delivered within 37 weeks' gestation. This entails rest in hospital until the bleeding has stopped. The RCOG[26] suggest that women in the third trimester should be hospitalised until delivery if major placenta praevia has been diagnosed. Enkin et al.[2] state that the two randomised trials comparing in-patient and out-patient care for known placenta praevia have not been large enough to permit definite conclusions about safety. Blood must be available should the mother bleed again and need a transfusion.

In-patient treatment includes correction of anaemia in the mother and serial ultrasound scans for foetal well-being. Anti-D and/or steroids should be administered (as in placental abruption) and psychological care must be considered. The mother may become institutionalised and miserable with prolonged hospitalisation. She may be separated from other children and need help in organising their care. She may need parentcraft education and a visit to the neonatal unit. A date set for her delivery will give her something positive to focus on.

Possible complications

Postpartum haemorrhage

Following delivery of a woman with placenta praevia or abruption uncontrollable bleeding may occur despite administration of oxytocics (*see* Chapter 10 for further details).

Coagulation defects

The trigger for disseminated intravascular coagulation (DIC) seems to be the entry of tissue thromboplastin or endotoxin into the circulation, inducing thrombin activation. A consumption coagulopathy occurs where fibrinogen, coagulation factors and circulating platelets are depleted. The result is haemostatic failure with microvascular bleeding and an increased blood loss. DIC can arise from placental abruption and haemorrhagic shock. (*See* Chapter 10 for further discussion of DIC.)

Anaemia

A result of excessive blood loss, this may require correction by blood transfusion or oral iron therapy. The RCOG[26] recommends that possible blood transfusion requirements are discussed with all women with placenta praevia and their partners prior to delivery to ensure that any objections or queries are dealt with effectively. Bonner[18] suggests that every unit should establish specific protocols for the management of women who refuse blood.

Infection

Infection may be acquired through low resistance caused by shock, anaemia or through increased interventions.

Renal failure

Renal failure may occur as a result of severe shock.

Hysterectomy

This can result from uncontrollable haemorrhage, particularly as a result of Couvelaire uterus or coagulation defects.

Sheehan's syndrome

Anterior pituitary necrosis or Sheehan's syndrome is a rare complication of prolonged shock. It can result in failure of lactation, amenorrhoea, hypothyroidism and adrenocortical insufficiency following the pregnancy.[18]

Foetal hypoxia

Foetal hypoxia may occur as a result of premature placental separation.

Premature delivery and resulting sequelae

Any delivery occurring between 24 and 37 weeks' gestation as a result of placental abruption or placenta praevia will require varying degrees of input from the neonatal unit. Long term follow-up may ensue and need input from the community and social services.

Foetal death

Death of the foetus is rare and more common in abruption (*see* above).

Adverse psychological effects

Such effects, as for example, postnatal depression or post traumatic stress syndrome could occur as a result of prolonged periods of hospitalisation, a traumatic delivery or negative foetal outcome. Midwives can help by generally debriefing and providing support if the baby is in the neonatal unit. It may be necessary to refer the mother for bereavement counselling and she may wish to receive advice on the risks for subsequent pregnancies (for example, the recurrence rate for placenta praevia is 4–8%).

Placenta accreta

This and its more advanced forms, increta and percreta, may occur in subsequent pregnancies. In such cases the placenta has become morbidly adherent to the uterine wall. This can occur when a woman has had a previous caesarean section.[27] Ziadeh et al.[27] carried out a retrospective review of case records to determine the relationship between previous caesarean section and subsequent development of placenta praevia with accreta. They found a high association between anterior placenta praevia, placenta accreta and previous caesarean section, which was enhanced with the increasing number of previous caesarean sections.

Check list: what to do when an antepartum haemorrhage occurs

In hospital some of the actions below will be done simultaneously because many personnel may be involved. Antepartum haemorrhage requires immediate action.

- Assess clinical situation.
- Perform cardiopulmonary resuscitation if necessary.
- Establish venous access and administer fluids.
- Arrange transfer to hospital by ambulance.
- Ensure appropriate personnel assembled.
- Continuous assessment of maternal condition.
- Replace blood loss as necessary.

- Assess foetal condition.
- Collect blood samples.
- Give analgesia as necessary.
- Deliver baby (if necessary) after mother stabilised.
- Documentation: time, action, reaction.
- Continual explanation and calm attitude.

Conclusion

It must be stressed that in all cases of antepartum haemorrhage, effective communication and accurate record keeping are important.

The continual training and updating of staff who may be involved in the management and treatment of antepartum haemorrhage at home or in hospital should be organised regularly. Because antepartum haemorrhage is a thankfully rare occurrence, training should be done in a memorable and interesting way.

Long[28] has observed that learners tend to feel anxious about being faced with a clinical situation with which they feel unable to cope. She suggests that they learn more effectively from guided study on the subject of antepartum haemorrhage with scenarios to work through in small groups to prepare them for a clinically focused session.

References

1 Konje J and Taylor D (1999) Bleeding in late pregnancy. In: D James, P Steer, C Weiner and B Gonik (eds) *High Risk Pregnancy Management Options*. WB Saunders, London.

2 Enkin M, Keirse M, Neilson JP et al. (eds) (2000) *A Guide to Effective Care in Pregnancy and Childbirth* (3e). Oxford University Press, Oxford.

3 Lewis G (ed) (2001) *Why Mothers Die 1997–1999: the fifth report of the confidential enquiries into maternal deaths in the United Kingdom*. RCOG Press, London.

4 Obed JY and Adewole IF (1996) Antepartum haemorrhage: the influence of first trimester uterine bleeding. *W African J Med.* **15** (1): 61–3.

5 Macones GA, Sehdev HM, Parry S et al. (1997) The association between maternal cocaine use and placenta praevia. *Am J Obstet Gynecol.* **1777** (5): 1097–110.

6 Ananth CV, Smulian JC, Vintzileos et al. (1997) The association of placenta previa with history of caesarian delivery and abortion: a metaanalysis. *Am J Obstet Gynecol.* **177** (5): 1070–8.

7 McMahon MJ, Li R, Schenck AP et al. (1997) Previous caesarian birth. *J Repro Med.* **42** (7): 409–12.

8 Hendricks MS, Chow YH, Bhagavath B et al. (1999) Previous caesarian section and abortion as risk factors for developing placenta praevia. *J Obstet Gynaecol Res.* **25** (2): 137–42.

9 Abu-Heija AT, El-Jallad F and Ziadeh S (1999) Placenta praevia: effect of age, gravidity, parity and previous caesarian section. *Gynaecol Obstet Invest.* **47** (1): 6–8.

10 Andres RL (1996) The association of cigarette smoking with placenta praevia and abruptio placentae. *Seminars Perinatol.* **20** (2): 154–9.

11 Ananth CV, Savitz DA, Bowes WA et al. (1997) Influence of hypertensive disorders and cigarette smoking on placental abruption and uterine bleeding during pregnancy. *Br J Obstet Gynaecol.* **104**: 572–8.

12 Ananth CV, Smulian JC and Vintzileos AM (1999) Incidence of placental abruption in relation to cigarette smoking and hypertensive disorders during pregnancy: a metaanalysis of observational studies. *J Obstet Gynaecol.* **4**: 662–8.

13 Bewley C (1994) Coping with domestic violence in pregnancy. *Nurs Standard.* **8** (50): 25–8.

14 O'Shea L (1996) Domestic violence in pregnancy. *Mod Midwife.* **6** (3): 10–12.

15 James-Hanman D and Long L (1994) Crime prevention: an issue for midwives? *Br J Midwif.* **2** (1): 29–32.

16 O'Donogue D (1993) Violence against wives. *Br J Midwif.* **1** (6): 284–7.

17 Baskett TF (1999) *Essential Management of Obstetric Emergencies.* Clinical Press, Bristol.

18 Bonner J (2000) Massive obstetric haemorrhage. In: S Arulkumaran (ed) *Emergencies in Obstetrics and Gynaecology.* Baillière Tindall, London.

19 Mabie W (1992) Placenta praevia. *Clin Perinatol.* **19** (2): 425–35.

20 Lam CM, Wong SF, Chow KM et al. (2000) Women with placenta praevia and antepartum haemorrhage have a worse outcome than those who do not bleed before delivery. *J Obstet Gynaecol.* **20** (1): 27–31.

21 Bendetti T (1996) Obstetric haemorrhage. In: S Gabbe, J Niebyl and J Simpson (eds) *Obstetrics: normal and problem pregnancies* (3e). Churchill Livingstone, New York.

22 Chilaka VN, Konje JC, Clarke S et al. (2000) Practice observed: is speculum examination on admission a necessary procedure in the management of all cases of antepartum haemorrhage? *J Obstet Gynaecol.* **20** (4): 396–8.

23 Department of Health (1998) *Why Mothers Die: report on confidential enquiries into maternal death in the United Kingdom 1994–1996.* The Stationery Office, London.

24 Crowley P (2001) Prophylactic steroids for preterm birth. *Cochrane Database of System Rev.* **2**.

25 Sunna E and Ziadeh S (1999) Transvaginal and transabdominal ultrasound for the diagnosis of placenta praevia. *J Obstet Gynaecol.* **19** (2): 152–4.

26 Paterson-Brown S (2000) Placenta praevia: diagnosis and management. RCOG Press, London.

27 Ziadeh SM, Abu-Heija AT and El-Jallad MF (1999) Placental praevia and accreta: an analysis of two years' experience. *J Obstet Gynaecol.* **19** (6): 584–6.

28 Long L (2000) Antepartum haemorrhage: teaching to enhance practice. *Pract Midwife.* **3** (5): 32–5.

CHAPTER 6

Malpresentations and malpositions

Joanne Chadwick

Malpresentation is a broad term used to describe any foetal presentation other than the vertex.[1] It includes non-cephalic (breech), non-vertex cephalic (face and brow) and non-longitudinal (transverse, oblique) lies.

Malposition is a term used to describe a presentation by the head where it is in an abnormal position, such that the diameter of the skull in relation to the pelvic opening is greater than normal. It includes occipitoposterior positioning which is dealt with on pages 76–9.

It is vital that the midwife is aware that these situations frequently result in prolonged and/or obstructed labour, and emergency delivery. The highest standards of knowledge and practice may well help to negate potentially poor outcomes.

Breech presentation

Definition and incidence

Breech presentation is a longitudinal lie with the foetal buttocks in the lower pole of the uterus. The denominator is the sacrum and the presenting diameter is the bitrochanteric (10cm). At 28 weeks' gestation the incidence of breech is approximately 15%. Spontaneous version reduces this percentage to approximately 3–4% at term.[2,3]

Classification[4]

Frank breech

The breech presents with flexion at the hips and extension at the knees. This is the most common presentation with a rate of about 70% (see Figure 6.1a).

Complete (flexed) breech

Presentation with flexion at the hips and the knees with feet beside the buttocks (see Figure 6.1b).

Footling breech

One or both feet are presenting with extension at the hip(s) and knee(s) (see Figure 6.1c).

Kneeling breech

Presentation with one or both hips extended. There is also flexion at the knees. The knee is the presenting part (see Figure 6.1d).

Predisposing factors and underlying pathophysiology

Breech presentation carries higher rates of perinatal mortality and morbidity than cephalic

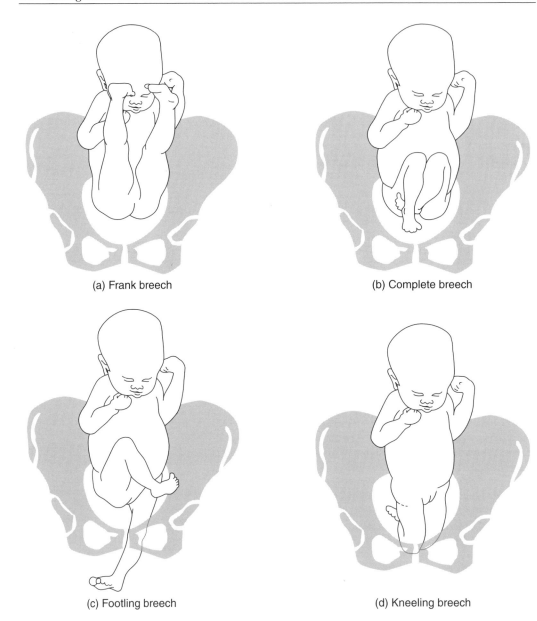

(a) Frank breech

(b) Complete breech

(c) Footling breech

(d) Kneeling breech

Figure 6.1 Classification of breech presentations

presentation.[5] Factors which may increase the incidence of breech include prematurity or intrauterine growth restriction. Before 34 weeks' gestation the foetus has more room to manoeuvre *in utero*. Both factors can result in the birth of a low birth weight baby which is in itself an indicator for poor perinatal outcome.[6]

Congenital malformations such as hydrocephaly also predispose to breech presentation. In such cases the foetal head is thought to be better accommodated in the fundus of the uterus. The foetus also has more room to move when the uterus is distended as in the case of poly-hydramnios. This condition must also alert the midwife to the increased risk of cord prolapse on rupture of the membranes.[7] Conversely, oligo-hydramnios may predispose to breech where, because of the small amount of fluid, foetal movement is restricted and the foetus is 'trapped' in the presentation assumed in the second trimester.[4]

The incidence of prolapsed cord is increased when the foetus is small (often premature or growth restricted) or the presenting breech is ill-fitting, but differs with each type of breech. With a frank breech the incidence is approximately 0.5% which is similar to the rate found in cephalic presentations. The rate increases to 5% for complete breech presentations and 15% for footling and knee presentations.[8,9] (*See* Chapter 9 for further information on cord prolapse.)

Multiple pregnancy carries an increased risk of breech because the space for one or more foetuses to turn is reduced and multiple preg-nancy is in itself a risk for preterm labour.[10]

Maternal factors thought to influence the incidence of breech presentation include any space-occupying uterine abnormalities. Examples include the presence of a septum or partial septum, or in rare cases the presence of uterine neoplasms such as leimyomata. Similarly, the presence of uterine fibroids and placental im-plantation in either the cornual-fundal region or in the lower uterine segment (placenta praevia) is thought to play a part in the aetiology of breech presentation. All these anomalies reduce uterine space for foetal movement.[4]

Research carried out in the USA cites maternal diabetes, older maternal age, smoking during pregnancy, primiparity and late or no prenatal care as all carrying an increased risk of breech presentation.[11] The authors discuss the possibility that several different factors and biological mech-anisms interact to increase the rate of breech.

Consideration should also be given to the fact that some women deliver all their children as breeches suggesting that their pelvic shape is better suited to a breech.[4] Research has indicated that recurring breech presentation represents a slightly lower risk of adverse perinatal outcome.[12] This may be due in part to more vigilant antenatal care. Although pelvic classification is controversial, obstetric texts frequently refer to an increased risk of breech with some pelvic shapes.[13] Examples include the platypelloid (anteroposteriorly flat) and android (heart-shaped); both these conditions make cephalic pelvic entry more difficult than in pelves with more favourable configurations.

Reducing the incidence of breech

Posture

Much has been written regarding the use of the knee–chest position as a means of encouraging spontaneous version from breech to cephalic presentation. Evidence from a Cochrane review describes how uncontrolled trials encourage women to adopt the knee–chest position for vary-ing time periods in late pregnancy. The review concludes that these studies show no significant benefit for breech version.[14] Smith et al.[15] reported no benefits in the use of postural management and saw no reason to recommend it. However, mid-wifery care emphasises psychological as well as physical benefits and so where no adverse conse-quences have been proved, the active involve-ment of the mother may well be beneficial to her.

Complementary therapies

There is some evidence that an acupuncture technique using moxibustion can be used to turn breech presentations and women may choose to access these services.[16]

External cephalic version

Current policy in many developed countries advises that when an uncomplicated breech presentation arises in the third trimester, external cephalic version should be attempted.[13] This pro-cedure has grown in popularity with the avail-ability of ultrasound, electronic foetal monitoring and effective tocolytic agents. Such interventions have been scrutinised by many randomised con-trolled trials and have yielded overwhelming evidence that there is a significant reduction in the risk of caesarean section in women under-going this procedure without any increased risk to the foetus. This procedure should therefore be offered to all women with an uncomplicated breech at term.[17,18]

Signs and symptoms

Abdominal palpation

Any history of previous breech presentation or the presence of any of the predisposing factors mentioned above should alert the midwife to the possibility of breech presentation.

On palpation, the lie is longitudinal and uterine size may palpate larger than expected from the dates. This is due to the fact that the breech may not have entered the pelvis. Using a Pawlik's grip, the head is located in the fundus and felt as a round hard mass which may move independently of the back by ballotting it with one or both hands.[7] Both poles of the foetus may be grasped simultaneously to aid diagnosis and if the entire breech is moveable above the pelvis it may be assumed that the foetal pelvis has not passed through the maternal pelvic inlet. Typically the foetal back is felt on one side of the abdomen and the foetal small parts on the other. Mothers with breech presentation often complain of discomfort under the ribs and heartburn caused by the proximity of the foetal head.[13]

Auscultation

Foetal heart sounds are often heard best at or above the umbilicus and laterally on the side of the foetal back.

Vaginal examination

The smooth head with its landmarks is absent. The presenting part is often high, is soft and irregular, and sometimes the anal orifice can be felt. If indistinguishable landmarks can be felt, in a breech they will be in a line (e.g. foetal ischial tuberosities and the anus).[19] After rupture of the membranes, fresh meconium can be noted especially on the examining finger following identification of the anus and this is diagnostic.[7] The midwife may also feel a foot or in rare circumstances, a knee. However, vaginal diagnosis of breech, particularly in early labour, is difficult and mistakes can be made.

Mechanism of labour: left sacro-anterior (LSA)

- Longitudinal lie.

- Attitude of flexion.

- Breech presentation.

- Position LSA.

- Denominator is the sacrum.

- The presenting part is the anterior left buttock.

- Engagement takes place when the bitrochanteric diameter has passed through the inlet of the pelvis.

- Descent takes place with increasing compaction. Since the breech is a less efficient dilator than the head, descent is usually slow (a sign that should alert the midwife when presentation is unsure).

- Flexion: lateral flexion takes place at the waist. The anterior hip becomes the leading part.

- Internal rotation of the buttocks: the anterior buttock reaches the resistance of the pelvic floor and rotates forwards to lie underneath the symphysis pubis.

- Lateral flexion of the baby: the anterior buttock impinges under the symphysis pubis, lateral flexion occurs and the posterior buttock is born. The buttocks then fall towards the anus and the anterior buttock is born (*see* Figure 6.2).

- The anterior buttock restitutes to the right.

- The shoulders enter the pelvis in the left oblique. The anterior shoulder rotates forward under the symphysis pubis. The posterior shoulder sweeps the perineum and is born (*see* Figure 6.3).

- As the shoulders are at the outlet the head enters the pelvis. It enters with the sagittal suture in the transverse diameter of the brim. The occiput meets the pelvic floor and rotates forward so that the sagittal suture is in the anteroposterior diameter.

- The sacrum rotates towards the pubis so the back is anterior.

- As the nape of the neck pivots under the symphysis, the chin, mouth, nose, forehead and occiput are born by flexion (*see* Figure 6.4).

Breech delivery

The first action of a midwife when confronted by an unexpected breech must be to call for help.[20] This would be either for medical assistance within a hospital setting or for emergency services in the community. Professional backup is imperative in both situations.

Position for delivery should be discussed with the woman. The most common position is

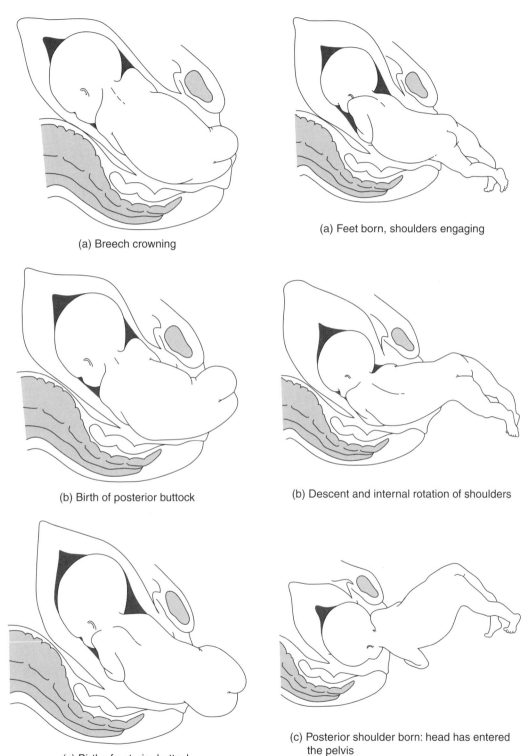

(a) Breech crowning

(a) Feet born, shoulders engaging

(b) Birth of posterior buttock

(b) Descent and internal rotation of shoulders

(c) Birth of anterior buttock

(c) Posterior shoulder born: head has entered the pelvis

Figure 6.2 Birth of the buttocks

Figure 6.3 Birth of the shoulders

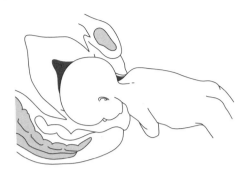

(a) Descent of head

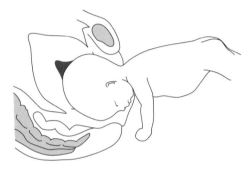

(b) Internal rotation of head

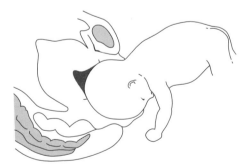

(c) Flexion of the head: birth of face

Figure 6.4 Birth of the head

semi-recumbent with space at the end of the bed to allow the baby to hang. Upright positions are controversial, but some midwives will suggest a position on hands and knees.[21]

Full dilatation of the cervix must be confirmed before encouraging the woman to push. This will prevent the head from becoming trapped within a partially dilated cervix. If this occurs, a retractor or finger can be used to push aside the cervix to clear an airway in the vagina for the baby's nose or mouth.[4] Delivery must then be expedited.

The baby's legs should deliver spontaneously, but if necessary they can be assisted by placing two fingers along the length of one thigh with the fingertips in the popliteal fossa. Each leg is then flexed across the body and down.

Once the baby has birthed to the umbilicus and the legs have been delivered, a loop of cord may be brought down to reduce cord tension although this is rarely necessary. The baby's body should be wrapped in a warm towel to prevent heat loss and stimulation of respiration.

The midwife can assess the position of the baby's arms by placing fingers on its chest. If she can feel elbows, the arms are flexed and should deliver with the next contraction. However, if the arms are extended the Løvset manoeuvre is necessary to continue the delivery. If traction has been used during the delivery, it is likely the arms will be extended. This is one reason to avoid traction and indeed any unnecessary handling during a breech delivery.

Løvset manoeuvre

Holding the baby at the hip bones with the thumbs over the sacrum, downward traction must be applied in combination with rotation. Care must be taken to always keep the foetal back towards the mother's front (i.e. the foetal back must be uppermost if the woman is in a semi-recumbent position). The baby is then rotated 180 degrees so as to splint the posterior arm across the baby's face and change it to an anterior position. If the arm does not then deliver spontaneously, the midwife should draw it gently down over the chest by flexing the elbow with her finger. The baby is then rotated back in the opposite direction and the second arm is delivered (*see* Figure 6.5).

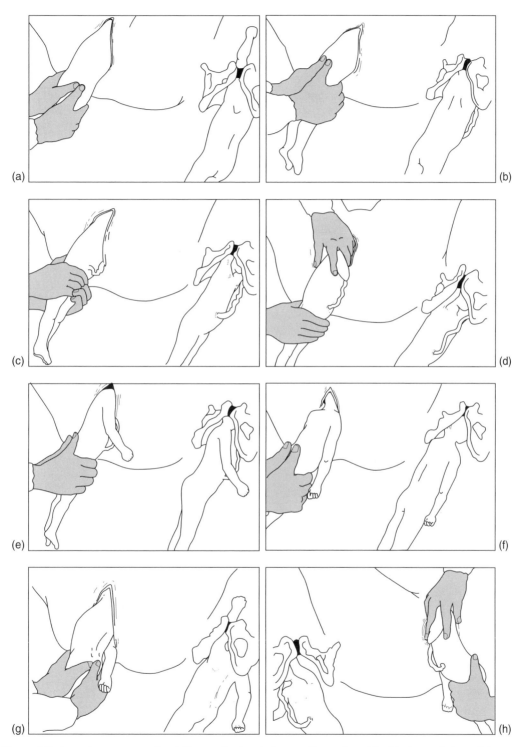

Figure 6.5 Løvset manoeuvre for delivery of extended arms. Reproduced by kind permission of the publisher, Churchill Livingstone, from Bennett R and Brown K (eds) (1999) *Myles' Textbook for Midwives* (13e), p. 531.

Delivery of the head

The head must be allowed to move through the pelvis in a transverse position until it rotates spontaneously to bring the occiput under the symphysis pubis with the back anterior. The head can then be delivered by one of two manoeuvres.

Burns Marshall manoeuvre

With the baby's back towards the mother's front (i.e. the baby's back is uppermost if the woman is semi-recumbent), the baby can be allowed to hang without support. This brings the head down onto the perineum. After one to two minutes the hairline will appear and the sub-occipital region can be felt. The midwife must grasp the baby's ankles and while maintaining traction, pivot the sub-occipital region through an arc of 180 degrees until the mouth and nose are free at the vulva. This is done slowly to prevent sudden changes in pressure to the head and the perineum is guarded to prevent sudden escape of the head. Care must also be taken not to overstretch or compress the baby's spine. As the face is born, suction is applied to clear the airway (*see* Figure 6.6).

Mauriceau-Smellie-Veit manoeuvre

The midwife should support the baby's body on her arm with her middle fingers placed on the baby's malar bones. This pulls the jaw downwards and increases flexion. The midwife should then place her other hand across the baby's shoulders with her middle fingers on the occiput to increase flexion. The head is drawn out until the sub-occipital region appears and the head is pivoted around the symphysis pubis (*see* Figure 6.7). This manoeuvre is also used when the foetal head is extended and descent is delayed.

Emergency breech extraction

This is carried out rarely and only as an emergency procedure to achieve immediate delivery of the baby when there is severe foetal distress or to deliver a second twin in a transverse or oblique lie after internal podalic version.

A hand must be placed into the uterus and if possible both feet grasped. The legs must be pulled down and the head pressed upwards with the outside hand. Traction must be maintained on the delivered legs until the breech is fixed (*see* Figure 6.8). Traction takes the place of

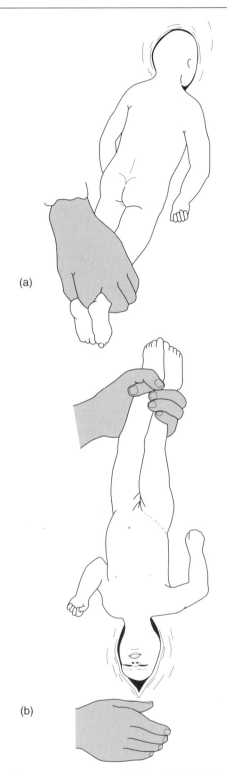

(a)

(b)

Figure 6.6 Burns Marshall method of delivering the after-coming head of a breech presentation

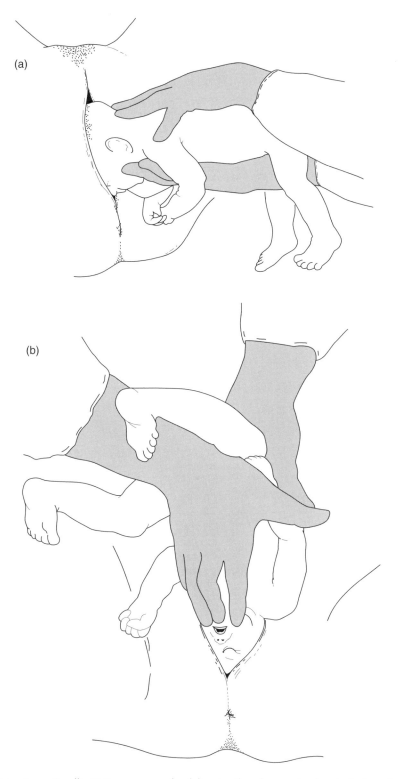

Figure 6.7 Mauriceau-Smellie-Veit manoeuvre for delivering the after-coming head of a breech presentation

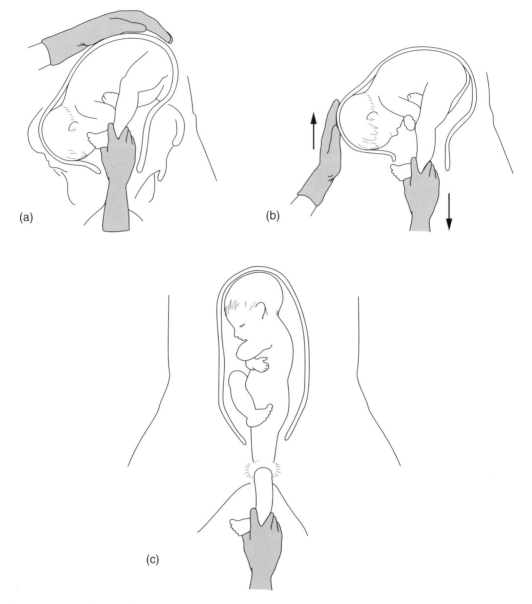

(a)

(b)

(c)

Figure 6.8 Breech extraction

contractions and the breech can then be delivered by the methods set out above.[22] As the arms will be extended following traction, Løvset's manoeuvre will be necessary to deliver the arms.

The breech delivery at home

There is a paucity of recent literature outlining risk and outcomes for planned breech births taking place at home. Existing studies indicate that risk to mother and baby may increase.[23] However, choice of venue is something all mothers should have, having first been guided and informed by up-to-date and sound evidence. In addition, choice must include different birth options and settings within the hospital environment.

Breech birth at home is fast becoming a rarity, as rising caesarean section rates reduce opportunities for midwives and doctors to gain skills in the delivery of vaginal breeches.[24,25] This recent trend deskills midwives as they lose not only the opportunity for hands-on experience, but also opportunities to observe vaginal breech delivery. However, as emphasised by the *Confidential Enquiry into Stillbirths and Deaths in Infancy*,[26] all midwives must maintain a good knowledge of breech delivery procedures as the chance of an undiagnosed and therefore unexpected breech presentation in second stage does exist.

Priorities for the midwife are to obtain help, maintain a calm environment and prepare for neonatal resuscitation starting with suction on delivery of the face. The environment must be kept warm to prevent neonatal hypothermia and ensuing hypoglycaemia. Early feeding is highly desirable.

The breech delivery in hospital

The same priorities as above apply. However, preparing for a breech delivery in hospital is now usually associated with preparation for surgery.

Although it is not within the scope of this chapter to discuss the evidence on choice of mode of breech delivery, it is important to note current trends based on research. Literature examining outcomes following vaginal versus caesarean breech delivery is abundant, but often contradictory. The most recent results from an international randomised controlled trial attest to the significantly lower rates of perinatal mortality, neonatal mortality and serious neonatal morbidity when planned caesarean section is carried out as opposed to vaginal birth.[27] No differences are noted in terms of serious maternal morbidity and the primary recommendation is for breech presentations to be delivered by caesarean section. This trial is not beyond criticism and already many questions regarding the protocol have been asked, for example about the positions that the women in the vaginal mode group were encouraged to adopt.[28] However, this study will be very influential and will further increase the rate of caesarean sections carried out for breech presentations (now approximately 90% in developed countries).[5]

Delivery of preterm infants with breech presentation is also controversial because of conflicting evidence regarding long- and short-term neurological and physical outcomes.[29,30] These controversies emphasise that it is imperative for midwives to keep themselves well informed with up-to-date information.

Possible complications

Baby

- Fractures of the humerus, clavicle or femur.
- Dislocation of the hip or shoulder.
- Erb's palsy.
- Internal organ damage by rough or faulty handling (e.g. kidneys, liver, spleen).
- Dislocation of the neck.
- Spinal cord damage or spinal fracture.
- Intracranial haemorrhage.
- Soft tissue damage.
- Hypoxia, birth asphyxia. This may be due to cord compression, cord prolapse or premature placental separation.
- Long-term neurological damage.
- Cold injury and hypoglycaemia.
- Congenital dislocation of the hip, especially with extended breech. This is usually a complication of the presentation, not the birth process.

Mother

- Urethral trauma.
- Vaginal or perineal trauma.
- Risks associated with operative delivery.
- Psychological distress may lead to poor bonding, feeding problems, depression and traumatic stress disorder.[31]

Vaginal breech delivery checklist

- Abdominal palpation.
- Vaginal examination to assess cervical dilatation.
- Auscultation.
- Possible assistance in delivery of extended legs.
- Release loop of cord as necessary.

- Check for position of arms.

- Wrap the baby in a towel to keep it warm.

- Keep the baby's back to the mother's front (i.e. back uppermost if woman is in semi-recumbent position).

- Løvset manoeuvre for arm or shoulder delivery if necessary.

- Allow descent of the head to sub-occipital region (avoidance of traction will ensure the head remains flexed).

- Slow delivery of the head using Burns Marshall or Mauriceau-Smellie-Veit manoeuvre.

- Suction and possible neonatal resuscitation.

- Maintain the baby's temperature.

- Early feeding.

- Paediatric assessment.

Conclusion

Breech presentation carries increased risks to mother and baby. Midwives must not only develop and maintain their skills for emergency delivery but also focus on the psychological impact of such a birth. Evidence-informed theory underpins practice and compassionate empathy underpins the art of midwifery. In combination, both allow midwives to provide the unique care that only they can give.

Transverse or oblique lie

The incidence of transverse lie is around 1:500. It occurs when the long axes of mother and foetus are at right angles to one another. The baby may lie directly in the transverse or in the oblique with head or breech in the iliac fossa (*see* Figure 6.9). The presenting part is frequently the shoulder.

Causes

Maternal causes include lax uterine muscles as seen in multiparity and uterine anomalies such as a bicornuate or sub-septate uterus. Placenta praevia and contracted pelvis also increase the risk.

Foetal causes include prematurity and poly-hydramnios, where the foetus has more room to change position, and multiple pregnancy.[32] Transverse lie is more common for the second baby in a twin delivery.

Signs and symptoms

Abdominal palpation

The uterus appears broad and no poles, for example the head or breech, are felt in the pelvis or fundus. If the shoulder becomes wedged in the pelvis, labour is obstructed and the uterine contractions may become tonic. The lower seg-ment may feel tender to the touch. If operative delivery is not expedited uterine rupture, death of the foetus and possible maternal death will ensue.[4]

Vaginal examination

Often little is felt on examination as the presenting part is high. If the midwife discovers a shoulder, she may feel a soft irregular mass or even the ribs. With a high presenting part the risk of cord prolapse is high. There is no mechanism for delivery of shoulder presentation.

Emergency management

- Call for medical assistance.

- Transfer to hospital.

- If the membranes rupture, check for cord prolapse (*see* Chapter 9).

- Prepare for delivery by caesarean section. In cases where facilities for caesarean do not exist or with a second twin delivery, internal podalic version may be attempted with the baby delivered as a footling breech. However, this is dangerous with high rates of neonatal mortality and morbidity.[4,13]

- Maternal risks include prolonged labour, fistula formation, infection from prolonged ruptured membranes, uterine rupture and psychological trauma.[33]

- Transverse lie is best dealt with antenatally where appropriate care can be planned to avoid the emergency situation.

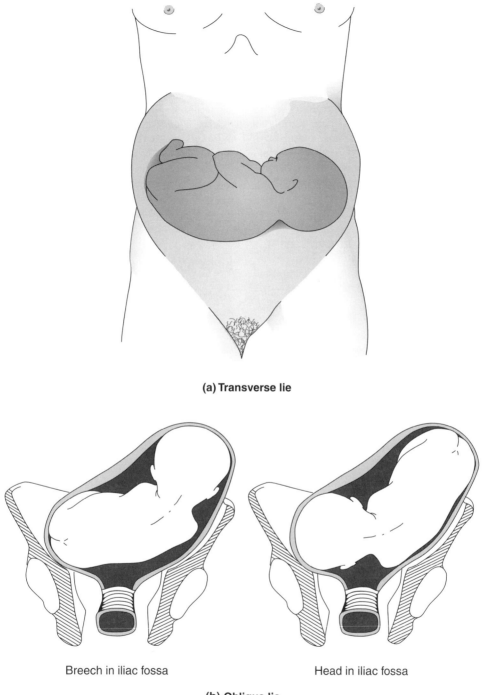

(a) Transverse lie

Breech in iliac fossa   Head in iliac fossa

(b) Oblique lie

Figure 6.9 Transverse and oblique lie

Occipitoposterior positioning

Definition and incidence

Occipitoposterior (OP) positioning occurs when the occiput is malpositioned in the posterior of the pelvis. More often than not, OP positions turn spontaneously. However in 10% of cases they do not and 5% of babies are delivered in the OP position.[34] As outcomes can differ with this position, labour is frequently prolonged and failure to progress may occur.

Predisposing factors and underlying pathophysiology

In most cases the aetiology of this malposition is unknown. However, women with a previous history of OP are more likely to suffer a repeat.[35] It has also been suggested that a contracted pelvis predisposes to OP with the occiput occupying the more spacious hindpelvis.[7] A recent study by Gardberg et al.[36] showed that 68% of persistent OP positions developed through a malrotation during labour from an initially anterior position.

Reducing the incidence of occipitoposterior

Randomised controlled trials to assess the impact of midwifery interventions on OP position have not been published. However, discussions of potential methods to help women are readily available. One suggestion is that the woman should assume a position on all fours with raised buttocks prior to and during labour. This position tilts the pelvis forward, maximising the angle between the spine and pelvis, and therefore the space available to enable the baby's head to engage more easily.[37]

During labour, the deflexed head in an OP position is often poorly applied to the cervix. Stimulation of oxytocin is reduced and labour is often slow. With modern management this type of labour is frequently augmented via amniotomy and Syntocinon®. El Halta[35] suggests that this is the worst thing that can be done as ruptured membranes encourage descent, limiting the

opportunity for rotation and predisposing to deep transverse arrest. With membranes intact, the mother can assume a position on all fours with the buttocks raised which encourages the head to rotate to an anterior position, with the amniotic fluid providing a cushion for the head.[35] Internal manual rotation to an anterior position has been suggested by Davis.[38] This technique involves placing fingers on the sagittal suture line, applying pressure to disengage the head and then turning the fingers to rotate the baby. This is not recommended for the inexperienced midwife, but may be more appropriate when recourse to medical assistance is not available and delivery needs to be expedited.

Signs and symptoms

Abdominal palpation

Occipitoposterior position should be considered if engagement has not occurred at term in the primiparous woman. This is because the OP position makes it more difficult for the foetus to negotiate the pelvis.

The foetal back may be difficult to find or is found to be in a lateral position. The foetal head is posterior-lateral and not engaged. A dip is often noted at the mother's umbilicus marking the space between the baby's arms and legs.[39] The foetal heartbeat is heard laterally or at the umbilicus.

Labour and vaginal examination

Labour may be slow or prolonged and the mother may complain of excessive back pain.[35] Early rupture of the membranes is common, especially if the presenting part is ill-fitting. OP is confirmed if the midwife locates the anterior fontanelle in the anterior during a vaginal examination. However, vaginal examination can be complicated by the presence of caput succedaneum and moulding.

Possible outcomes of labour

Long internal rotation

If engagement occurs in the transverse or right oblique diameter of the brim, descent occurs in the right oblique diameter as a right occipitoposterior position. Descent continues to the pelvic floor and progress depends on flexion of the head. If flexion increases and the occiput meets the resistance of the pelvic floor, it will first rotate anteriorly through 135 degrees to a direct occipito-anterior (OA) position and then birth occurs as in the usual OA position.

Short internal rotation

If the foetal head is deflexed and remains that way anterior rotation of the occiput may not occur. The sinciput reaches the resistance of the pelvic floor and rotates forwards. The occiput settles into the hollow of the sacrum and the foetal chest restricts flexion of the head. Maternal soft tissues are stretched more and the midwife may suspect this position if there is gaping of the vagina and dilatation of the anus while the foetal head is barely visible. Upward moulding and caput suc-cedaneum are evident and the baby is born face to pubis – persistent occipitoposterior (POP).

On delivery the sinciput will emerge under the symphysis and the midwife may support the head to prevent rapid expulsion of the occiput over the perineum. Management will depend on whether the midwife uses a hands-on or hands-poised method. Increased risk for perineal trauma must be anticipated in both cases.

Deep transverse arrest

As the head descends with a degree of flexion, the occiput begins to rotate forwards as in a long internal rotation. However, without complete flexion the occipitofrontal diameter becomes trapped between the bispinous diameter of the outlet. On vaginal examination, the sagittal suture is found in the transverse diameter usually with both fontanelles palpable. The foetal head does not advance. Medical assistance should be summoned and rotational forceps or manual rotation may be attempted. However, recent trends have ensured that most of these cases are delivered by caesarean section.

The use of rotational forceps by experienced clinicians has been shown to have similar outcomes to caesarean section.[40] However, the decrease in the use of forceps, especially rotational, in favour of vacuum extraction (ventouse) will result in a reduced number of experienced practitioners. If instrumental delivery is deemed to be difficult, the consensus is that caesarean delivery is preferable.[2]

Face presentation

This occurs in about 1:600 cases and the denominator is the mentum.[13] The face may be a primary presentation or result from an OP position. The latter is called a secondary face presentation and develops as contractions pro-mote extension of the head.

Vaginal examination

The presenting part is often high and facial features may be felt. The mouth and two malar prominences will be felt as a triangle.[19] Care must be taken not to damage the eyes.

Mechanism

Engagement is usually in the transverse diameter of the brim producing a right or left mentolateral position. Descent continues until the pelvic floor is reached and rotation occurs. The mentum leads and rotates forwards until it sits under the sym-physis. Descent increases extension of the face as the occiput is pushed towards the foetal back.

After anterior rotation and descent, the chin and mouth appear at the vulva. Then the nose, eyes, brow and occiput sweep the perineum and the head delivers by flexion. The chin then rotates to the side towards which it was originally directed and the shoulders are delivered as normal (see Figure 6.10). The face and oedema will be distorted.

In 75% of cases the face presents with the mentum anterior.[13] Unless the foetus is very small, delivery from the mentoposterior position will not occur. The foetal neck is shorter than the maternal sacrum and cannot stretch to fill the hollow of the sacrum.

Delivery

Over 50% of face presentations are not diag-nosed until the second stage and intervention is not warranted unless there is severe foetal dis-tress, arrest of dilatation or arrest of descent. The midwife can be reassured that the majority of mentoanterior presentations will deliver vaginally. However, medical assistance for caesarean section and neonatal resuscitation should be on stand-by.[41]

Brow presentation

When the foetal head is partially extended, the presenting diameter is the mentovertical (13.5 cm).

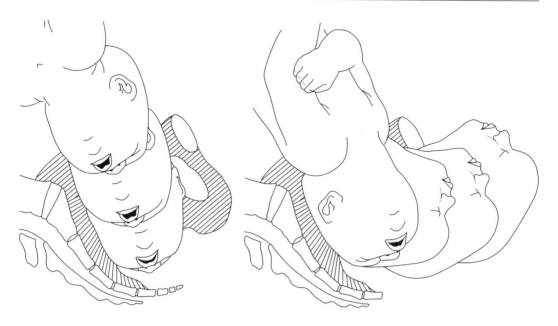

Figure 6.10 Face presentation (mentoanterior) and delivery

This exceeds all diameters within the pelvis. Thankfully, this presentation is rare with a reported incidence of about 1:700.[42] The majority of cases occur without reason although the presentation is associated with contracted pelves and an OP position.[42]

Vaginal examination

The presenting part is often high, the anterior fontanelle may be felt on one side of the pelvis and the orbital ridges on the other. If arrest of the brow occurs, labour will become obstructed.

Delivery

Vaginal delivery is rare and caesarean section should be anticipated. However, if the brow descends to meet the pelvic floor, the maxilla rotates forwards and the head is born like a POP presentation. Continued extension may convert the brow to a face presentation and occasionally flexion may convert the brow to a vertex presentation with resulting vaginal delivery. This has been reported in study groups with rates as high as 25%.[42]

Occipitoposterior delivery at home

Labour with this position has been shown to have a variety of outcomes. Vigilance on the part of the midwife is vital and any sign of prolonged labour and delay at any point should alert her to the possibility of malposition or malpresentation. Monitoring progress and detailed vaginal examinations are vital and any concerns should warrant the summons of medical assistance. Encouraging changes of position may offer solutions and psychological support for the mother is paramount. Preparation for neonatal resuscitation should be made.

Occipitoposterior delivery in hospital

Care and management in the home or hospital is similar. Aware of possible outcomes, the midwife must act as advocate for the mother, and ensure that rapid interventions are not imposed without full discussion and examination of evidence. OP presentation is still a cephalic presentation and is within the scope of midwifery practice.

Possible complications of malposition

Baby

- Hypoxia resulting from prolonged labour or cord prolapse (predisposed by a high head with ill-fitting presenting part).
- Risk of infection if there is prolonged rupture of membranes.
- Cerebral haemorrhage from unfavourable upward moulding.
- Facial bruising with face presentation.
- Hypothermia and hypoglycaemia if hypoxic or if resuscitation has been required.

Mother

- Prolonged labour.
- Exhaustion, dehydration and ketosis.
- Perineal lacerations and trauma.
- Trauma from operative delivery.
- Risk of infection if prolonged rupture of membranes has taken place.
- Psychological trauma.

Occipitoposterior delivery checklist

Outcomes

- Long rotation to occipitoanterior and normal delivery.
- Short rotation to POP with face to pubis delivery.
- Deep transverse arrest.
- Conversion to face presentation (mentoanterior can deliver vaginally, mentoposterior unlikely).
- Conversion to brow presentation (may convert to face or vertex; if not, vaginal delivery unlikely).
- Call for medical assistance if foetal delay or arrest, or non-vertex presentation occurs.
- Medical intervention for instrumental or operative delivery.

Actions

- Prepare for neonatal resuscitation.
- Keep the baby warm.
- Early feeding.
- Paediatric assessment.

Conclusion

Malpresentations and malpositions are often part of the birth process. Midwives should always expect the unexpected even while promoting birth as a normal physiological and psychosocial event in the life of the woman and her family. Safe practice based on sound theory is vital and such knowledge must include all aspects of the birth process. Practice, judgement and skills need to be constantly reviewed and updated.

References

1 Kopelman JN, Maslow AS, Markenson GR and Foley KS (1996) Malpresentation. In: JT Repke (ed) *Intrapartum Obstetrics*. Churchill Livingstone, New York.
2 Hofmeyr GJ (2000) Breech presentation and abnormal lie in late pregnancy. In: M Enkin, MJNC Keirse, J Neilson et al. (eds) *A Guide to Effective Care in Pregnancy and Childbirth*. Oxford University Press, Oxford.
3 Cheng M and Hannah M (1993) Breech delivery at term: a critical review of the literature. *Obstet Gynaecol.* **82**: 605–18.
4 Oxorn-Foote H (1986) *Human Labor and Birth* (5e). Appleton-Century-Crofts, New York.
5 Sanders NJS (1996) Breech delivery in the UK at the end of this century. *Contemp Rev Obstet Gynaecol.* **8** (2): 82–5.
6 McCloskey L and Wise PH (1998) Maternal and infant health in the United States: implications for women's health. In: H Wallace et al. (eds) *Health and Welfare for Families in the 21st Century*. Jines and Bartlett, New York.
7 Coates T (1999) Malpositions of the occiput and malpresentations. In: VR Bennett and LK Brown (eds) *Myles Textbook for Midwives* (13e). Churchill Livingstone, Edinburgh.
8 Collea JV, Rabin SC, Weghorst GR et al. (1978) The randomised management of term frank breech presentation: vaginal delivery

versus caesarian section. *Am J Obstet Gynaecol.* **131**: 186.

9 Barrett JMF (1991) Funic reduction for the management of umbilical cord prolapse. *Am J Obstet Gynecol.* **165**: 654.

10 Lewis TLT and Chamberlain GVP (eds) (1996) Fetal malposition and malpresentation. In: *Obstetrics by Ten Teachers* (15e). Edward Arnold, London.

11 Rayl J, Gibson PJ and Hickok DE (1996) A population-based case-controlled study of risk factors for breech presentation. *Am J Obstet Gynecol.* **174** (1): 28–32.

12 Albrechtsen S, Rasmussen S, Dalaker K et al. (1998) Perinatal mortality in breech presentation sibships. *Obstet Gynecol.* **92** (5): 775–80.

13 Cunningham FG, McDonald PC, Grant NF et al. (1996) *Williams Obstetrics* (20e). McGraw-Hill, New York.

14 Hofmeyr GJ (1999) Cephalic version by postural management for breech presentation. In: *The Cochrane Library* (Issue 3). Update Software, Oxford.

15 Smith C, Crowther C, Wilkinson C et al. (1999) Knee-chest postural management for breech at term: a randomised controlled trial. *Birth.* **26** (2): 71–5.

16 Budd S (1995) Acupuncture. In: D Tiran and S Mack (eds) *Complementary Therapies for Pregnancy and Childbirth*. Baillière Tindall, London.

17 Hofmeyr GJ (1999) External cephalic version for breech presentation at term. In: *The Cochrane Library* (Issue 1). Update Software, Oxford.

18 Clinical Audit Unit (1997) Breech presentation at term. In: *Effective Procedures in Maternity Care Suitable for Audit*. RCOG Press, London.

19 American Academy of Family Physicians (1996) *Advanced Life Support in Obstetrics (ALSO) Training Manual* (3e). American Academy of Family Practitioners, Newcastle upon Tyne.

20 United Kingdom Central Council for Nursing, Midwifery and Health Visiting (1998) *Midwives Rules and Code of Practice*. UKCC, London.

21 Cronk M (1998) Midwives and breech births. *Pract Midwife.* **1** (7): 44–5.

22 Miller AWF and Callander R (1989) Malposition and malpresentation. In: GVP Chamberlain (ed) *Obstetrics Illustrated* (4e). Churchill Livingstone, Edinburgh.

23 Mehl-Madrona L and Mehl-Madrona M (1997) Physician and midwife attended home births: effects of breech, twin and post-dates outcome data on mortality rates. *J Nurse-Midwif.* **42** (2): 91–8.

24 Irion O, Almagbaly PH and Morabia A (1998) Planned vaginal delivery versus elective caesarian section: a study of 705 singleton term breech presentations. *Br J Obstet Gynaecol.* **105** (7): 710–17.

25 Sharma JB, Newman MR, Boutchier JE et al. (1997) National audit on the practice and training in breech delivery in the UK. *Int J Gynaecol Obstet.* **59** (2): 103–8.

26 Maternal and Child Health Research Consortium (1998) *Confidential Enquiry into Stillbirths and Deaths in Infancy (Fifth Annual Report)*. Maternal and Child Health Research Consortium, London.

27 Hannah ME, Hannah WJ, Hewson SA et al. (2000) Planned caesarian section versus planned vaginal birth for breech presentation at term: a randomised multicentre trial. *Lancet.* **356**: 1375–83.

28 Gyte J and Frohlich J (2001) Commentary on 'Planned caesarian section versus planned vaginal birth for breech presentation at term: a randomised multicentre trial'. *MIDIRS Midwif Digest.* **11** (1): 80–3.

29 Wolf H, Schaap AP, Bruinse W et al. (1999) Vaginal delivery compared with caesarian section in early preterm breech delivery: a comparison of long-term outcome. *Br J Obstet Gynaecol.* **106** (5): 486–91.

30 Demol S, Bashir A, Furman B et al. (2000) Breech presentation is a risk for intrapartum and neonatal death in preterm deliveries. *Eur J Obstet Gynaecol Repro Biol.* **93** (1): 47–51.

31 Albrechtsen S, Rasmussen S, Dalaker K et al. (1998) Reproductive career after breech presentation: subsequent pregnancy rates, intrapregnancy interval and recurrence. *Obstet Gynecol.* **92** (3): 345–50.

32 Gemer O and Segal S (1994) Incidence and contribution of predisposing factors to transverse lie presentation. *Int J Gynaecol Obstet.* **44** (3): 219–21.

33 Arrowsmith S, Hamlin EC and Wall LL (1996) Obstructed labour injury complex: obstetric fistula formation and the multifaceted morbidity of maternal birth trauma in the developing world. *Obstet Gynaecol Surv.* **51** (9): 568–74.

34 Gardberg M and Tuppurainen M (1994) Effects of the persistent occipito-posterior presentation on the mode of delivery. *Geburtshilfe Perinatol.* **198**: 117.

35 El Halta V (1996) Posterior labour – a pain in the back: its prevention and cure. *Clarion.* **11** (1): 6–7, 12–13.

36 Gardberg M, Laakkonen ES and Levaara M (1998) Intrapartum sonography and persistent occiput posterior position: a study of 408 deliveries. *Obstet Gynecol.* **91** (5:1): 746–9.

37 Walmsley K (2000) Managing the occipito-posterior labour. *MIDIRS Midwif Digest.* **10** (1): 61–2.

38 Davis E (1997) *Heart and Hands: a midwife's guide to pregnancy and birth.* Celestial Arts, California.

39 Sutton J (2000) Occipito-posterior positioning and some ideas about how to change it. *Pract Midwife.* **3** (6): 20–2.

40 Jain V, Guleria K, Gopalan S et al. (1993) Mode of delivery in deep transverse arrest. *Int J Gynaecol Obstet.* **43** (2): 129–35.

41 O'Grady JP (1988) *Modern Instrumental Delivery.* Williams and Wilkins, Baltimore.

42 Abell DA (1973) Brow presentation. *S African Med J.* **47**: 13–15.

CHAPTER 7

Amniotic fluid embolism

Maureen Boyle

Amniotic fluid embolism is an obstetric emergency that is impossible to predict, offers minimal, if any, warning signs and usually has a tragic outcome. Eight deaths from amniotic fluid embolism were reported in the most recent *Report on Confidential Enquiries into Maternal Deaths*[1] proving that it continues to be a major cause of maternal mortality. Amniotic fluid embolism is difficult to diagnose, especially when the outcome is not fatal. Therefore the incidence rates have been quoted at anywhere from 1:8000 to 1:80 000, with a mortality rate of up to 90%, although one recent American study showed a low maternal mortality rate of 26.4%.[2,3]

An early description of amniotic fluid embolism was made in 1941 as 'maternal pulmonary embolism by amniotic fluid', after finding amniotic fluid in the pulmonary vessels at autopsy, following a collapse during delivery with symptoms mimicking pulmonary embolism.[4] Knowledge of the condition has only developed slowly since then, due to its rarity. However in 1988 a central registry recording women suffering from amniotic fluid embolism in the USA was set up and reports from this group have contributed to awareness.[5] In the UK, a similar registry was set up in 2000.[6]

Pathophysiology

Amniotic fluid can enter the maternal circulation through the endocervical veins and indeed may do so frequently without damage.[7] Obvious times of risk are during caesarean section or uterine rupture, but since amniotic fluid embolism can occur without these scenarios, it is also suggested that there may be small injuries during labour that allow the fluid access to maternal circulation. Amniotomy is an intervention that may cause injury and it has been reported that in the American Registry 78% of women with amniotic fluid embolism had ruptured membranes (two-thirds being artificial rupture of membranes (ARM)).[6] In 13% of cases only three minutes separated the ARM or insertion of intrauterine pressure catheters (IUPCs) and the maternal collapse. However, it is clear that in some cases the damage may occur spontaneously.

Although amniotic fluid can enter the maternal circulation without causing problems, in some women it seems an inflammatory response can develop causing a rapid collapse similar to anaphylaxis or septic shock.[8] One suggestion is that amniotic fluid in the maternal circulation could result in the release of a substance which leads to pulmonary vascular spasm, which in turn causes left ventricular failure.[9] This does not occur in all women, but why some are susceptible and others are not is unknown.

The volume of amniotic fluid entering the maternal circulation does not seem relevant, as embolism has been diagnosed during termination of early pregnancy, when there is only a very small amount of fluid present.[8]

Although the exact underlying pathophysiology and the reasons why any individual woman might be susceptible are not completely understood, the physical effects are clear. The pulmonary circulation is compromised, and left ventricular failure and coronary artery vasospasm causing myocardial ischaemia are involved.

Secondary coagulation problems affect about 40% of those who survive the initial event.[10] The cause of this coagulopathy is also not well understood, but it is known that amniotic fluid is a procoagulant.[11]

There have been reports of amniotic fluid embolism occuring later than would be expected, for example following caesarean section rather than during the procedure. It is suggested that such a delayed reaction may occur following a spinal anaesthesia if the amniotic fluid is present in dilated uterine veins and this is displaced when the block wears off and the venous tone is allowed to return.[12]

Diagnosis

Traditionally diagnosis of amniotic fluid embolism has only been made on post mortem examination when foetal cells or debris have been found during histological analysis of the maternal lungs.[13] Diagnosis has also been made in women who have survived, for example, following special staining of blood from the mothers' pulmonary vessels[2] or after finding foetal squames in sputum. Of course these tests are usually carried out only when the mother's physical condition is compromised.

Diagnosis of amniotic fluid embolism through analysis of maternal serum has been suggested. Research has been done into testing for the presence of elevated levels of sialyl Tn antigen, a constituent of amniotic fluid and meconium, and has demonstrated that this may be a possible test to detect amniotic fluid embolism.[14]

However most authorities agree that diagnosis should be made on the basis of clinical signs and symptoms. Clark[8] describes the sudden onset of a triad of symptoms, namely hypotension, hypoxia and coagulopathy as highly suspicious. Amniotic fluid embolism should always be suspected if a previously asymptomatic healthy woman develops cardiac or respiratory failure during labour, caesarean section or immediately after. It can also occur during termination of pregnancy.[1,15]

Signs and symptoms

The analysis of the American Registry showed that the symptoms of women diagnosed with amniotic fluid embolism were as follows, given in the order in which they most commonly occurred:[5]

- hypotension

- foetal distress
- pulmonary oedema
- cardiopulmonary arrest
- cyanosis
- coagulopathy
- respiratory distress
- convulsions
- uterine atony
- bronchospasm.

However in individual women, these symptoms can appear alone, in combination and of course in any order. 10–15% of women may have seizures as the first sign of amniotic fluid embolism, obviously causing the potential for confusion with eclampsia.[9]

Predisposing factors

(see Box 7.1 for a summary)

Induction with prostaglandins or oxytocin, or augmentation with oxytocin or ARM are often considered to be associated with amniotic fluid embolism. Of the eight deaths reported in the most recent *Report on Confidential Enquiries into Maternal Deaths*,[1] three of the women had had labour induced and two had received augmentation. In the previous report,[13] about half of the women who died from amniotic fluid embolism, either collapsed before labour commenced or laboured spontaneously. The role of induction and augmentation as a predisposing factor for amniotic fluid embolism is therefore far from clear.

Box 7.1: Possible predisposing factors

- 'Tumultuous' contractions.
- Age.
- Multiple pregnancy.
- Multiparity.
- Induction/augmentation.
- Invasive interventions in labour.

'Tumultuous' labour was decribed in 28% of women in one American report,[9] and abnormally strong contractions have also been noted by previous Confidential Enquiries in the UK.[13]

If the strength of contractions is considered to have influence over the occurrence of amniotic fluid embolism, multiparous women could be assumed to have very strong contractions and therefore be at increased risk. Out of 17 maternal mortalities for amniotic fluid embolism in the UK reported in the years 1994–96, nine women had a history of two or more previous deliveries.[13] However an association between parity and increased risk of amniotic fluid embolism was not found in the latest report.[1] Conversely, multiparity has been found to be a factor in 75–88% of cases in American studies.[3,5,9]

Multiple pregnancy has not been identified as a risk factor in Confidential Enquiry reports in the UK, although in the most recent report one woman was pregnant with twins.[1,13] However it has been noted in American studies.[3]

Prolonged labour has not been found to be a predisposing factor to amniotic fluid embolism.[16]

There is an association between amniotic fluid embolism and operative or instrumental deliveries, and with any invasive interventions such as amniotomy, insertion of IUPCs and amnioinfusion.

Amniotic fluid embolism is more common with increasing age. The *Report on Confidential Enquires into Maternal Deaths*[13] identified that in the years 1994–96 the mortality rate of women under 25 with amniotic fluid embolism was 0.4 in every million maternities, whereas the rate for those of 35–39 years of age was 10.4 and for those over 40 years, 37.0. In the most recent report increasing age was again noted to be relevant.[1] Increasing age has also been found to be a risk factor in a large American study, where the average age of those with amniotic fluid embolism was found to be 33 years.[3]

Although the roles of different risk factors are uncertain, it is relevant to note that only one woman with low parity and an uncomplicated pregnancy died from amniotic fluid embolism in the UK from 1994–96.[13] In 1997–99 two women with uncomplicated pregnancies died in the UK.[1]

Treatment

Since it is not yet possible to clearly identify those women who are at risk of amniotic fluid embolism or to prevent it, the focus must be on providing those women who collapse with prompt and competent first aid prior to a speedy transfer to where they can receive expert support and care, usually in an intensive care unit. This can improve their chances not only of survival, but of a complete recovery. General aims of treatment are given in Box 7.2:

Box 7.2: Treatment aims

• Circulatory support.

• Respiratory support.

• Correct coagulopathy.

Initial care

This will be the same whether at home or in hospital and includes the following:

• call for emergency help

• intravenous access and fluids

• ventilation: mouth to mouth, manual ventilation with an ambubag or intubation, depending on the site and availability of equipment or personnel

• cardiac massage as necessary.

Ongoing care

Following the arrival of help in hospital or the woman's arrival at hospital, the priorities of care given in Box 7.2 continue:

• administer fluids to maintain circulation (may be blood, fresh frozen plasma, cryoprecipitates, crystalloids or platelets depending on availability and the woman's need)

• monitor clotting and correct coagulopathy

• early endotrachael intubation[17]

• maintain oxygenation via intermittent positive pressure ventilation (IPPV) as necessary

• monitor condition with central venous pressure or arterial lines

- careful fluid balance and renal assessment

- administer drugs as necessary:

  - dopamine (increases cardiac output)
  - hydrocortisone (reduces inflammatory response)
  - sodium bicarbonate (corrects acidosis)
  - Syntocinon® infusion (if uterine atony).

Support and care for partners and others must not be neglected (*see* Chapter 2 for further discussion on this important matter) and consideration of psychological support for women who survive is necessary.

Complications

Of women who collapse with amniotic fluid embolism, 25–50% die within the first hour.[15] Of the eight women who died of amniotic fluid embolism in the UK from 1997–99, six died within four hours of their collapse. The most common short-term complication of amniotic fluid embolism is disseminated intravascular coagulation (DIC), arising in around half of those who survive more than one hour.[15] Many survivors have permanent neurological damage and neurologically intact survival has been estimated as only about 15%.[16]

If the woman is still pregnant when suffering the amniotic fluid embolism, the foetus may not survive. Estimates of foetal survival rates range from 39–80%. If the baby lives, neurological damage to the infant is common.[5]

Following recovery from an amniotic fluid embolism, a successful future pregnancy may be possible but the literature is very limited on this subject.[18]

Conclusion

It is not possible to clearly identify how to prevent amniotic fluid embolism. However it is clear that care needs to be taken in the use of prostaglandins and oxytocins, particularly in those women with other possible risk factors, for example age, parity and obstetric complications, and that other obstetric interventions, such as amniotomy, should be used only when necessary.

Confidential Enquiries reports have recommended that better treatment for those women who survive the initial event may help improve the outcome. However in the 1994–96 report only one case was identified as receiving substandard treatment following amniotic fluid embolism and in the latest report, although substandard features were identified in two cases, they were not thought to be critical to the outcome.[1,13]

Box 7.3: Key points of midwifery care

- Use midwifery skills to augment slow labour (e.g. support, mobilisation, comfort strategies, etc.) to avoid amniotomy and oxytocin use.

- Despite their common use, always treat prostaglandin and oxytocin with respect and monitor all women receiving these drugs carefully to avoid overstimulation. Use particular care when administering to older women, multiparous women or those with other complications.

- If a woman collapses at home or in hospital, prompt effective emergency support can improve her chance of complete recovery.

References

1 Lewis G (ed) (2001) *Why Mothers Die 1997–1999: the fifth report of the confidential enquiries into maternal deaths in the United Kingdom.* RCOG Press, London.

2 Locksmith G (1999) Amniotic fluid embolism. *Obstet Gynecol Clin N Am.* **26** (3): 435–44.

3 Gilbert W and Danielsen B (1999) Amniotic fluid embolism: decreased mortality in a population-based study. *Obstet Gynecol.* **93** (6): 973–7.

4 Steiner P and Lushbaugh C (1941) Maternal pulmonary embolism by amniotic fluid: as a cause of obstetric shock and unexpected deaths in obstetrics. *JAMA* **117** (15): 1245–54.

5 Clark S, Hankins G, Dudley D et al. (1995) Amniotic fluid embolism: analysis of the national registry. *Am J Obstet Gynecol.* **172** (4:1): 1158–69.

6 Tuffnell D and Johnson H (2000) Amniotic fluid embolism: the UK register. *Hosp Med.* **61** (8): 532–4.

7 Clark S, Pavlova Z and Greenspoon J (1986) Squamous cells in the maternal pulmonary circulation. *Am J Obstet Gynecol.* **154**: 104.

8 Clark S (1997) Amniotic fluid embolism: current concepts. *Contemp Rev Obstet Gynecol.* **9** (4): 297–301.

9 Martin R (1996) Amniotic fluid embolism. *Clin Obstet Gynecol.* **39** (1): 101–6.

10 Lau G and Chui P (1994) Amniotic fluid embolism: a review of 10 fatal cases. *Singapore Med J.* **35** (2): 180–3.

11 Lockwood C, Bach R, Guha A et al. (1991) Amniotic fluid contains tissue factor, a potent initiator of coagulation. *Am J Obstet Gynecol.* **165** (5:1): 1335–41.

12 Margarson M (1995) Delayed amniotic fluid embolism following cesarean section under spinal anaesthesia. *Anaesthesia.* **50** (9): 804–6.

13 Department of Health (1998) *Why Mothers Die: report on confidential enquiries into maternal deaths in the United Kingdom 1994–1996.* The Stationery Office, London.

14 Kobayashi H, Ohi H and Terao T (1993) A simple, noninvasive, sensitive method for diagnosis of amniotic fluid embolism by monoclonal antibody TKH–2 that recognizes NeuAca2–6GalNAc. *Am J Obstet Gynecol.* **168** (3:1): 848–53.

15 Baskett T (1999) *Essential Management of Obstetric Emergencies* (3e). Clinical Press, Bristol.

16 Hayashi R (2000) Obstetric collapse. In: LH Kean, PN Baker and DI Edelstone (eds) *Best Practice in Labor Ward Management.* WB Saunders, Edinburgh.

17 Benedetti T (1996) Obstetric haemorrhage. In: S Gabbe, J Niebyl and J Simpson (eds) *Obstetrics: normal and problem pregnancies* (3e). Churchill Livingstone, New York.

18 Clark (1992) Successful pregnancy outcomes after amniotic fluid embolism. *Am J Obstet Gynecol.* **167** (2): 511–12.

CHAPTER 8

Uterine inversion and uterine rupture

Debra Kroll and Michelle Lyne

Uterine inversion

Uterine inversion is a rare but life-threatening complication of the third stage of labour and is classified by time and severity.[1] The uterus can be described as inverted when the fundus has prolapsed into the body of the uterus and beyond. When this occurs immediate action must be taken to prevent maternal morbidity and mortality.

Uterine inversion has been cited as occurring at a rate of anything from 1:2000 to 1:50 000.[2] The widespread variation in this rate is dependent on third stage management and the level of reporting.[2,3]

Time

Acute inversion

This can occur during the third stage, when the placenta may or may not be attached, and up to 24 hours after delivery of the baby. It can be associated with cervical constriction and a cervical contraction ring may also form, which will impede replacement of the uterus.

Subacute inversion

This occurs 24 hours after delivery and up to 28 days postpartum. A cervical contraction ring is usually present.

Chronic inversion

This occurs after 28 days.[4,5,6,7,8]

Severity

This is determined by degrees.[6,7,9,10]

First degree (incomplete)

The fundus extends to, but not beyond, the cervix.

Second degree

The fundus protrudes through the cervix and past the cervical ring.

Third degree (complete)

The fundus extends to the perineum. If the fundus, cervix and vagina are visible this constitutes a uterine prolapse.

Aetiology

Uterine inversion can be iatrogenic, caused by mismanagement of the third stage of labour, including:

- early and excessive controlled cord traction before signs of placental separation

- controlled cord traction when the uterus is relaxed

- the use of fundal pressure with or without cord traction.

It can also occur spontaneously after rapid decompression of the uterus, as with the delivery of a macrosomic baby or twins or, rarely, following increased intra-abdominal pressure when the uterus can be forced down and out as a result of coughing and vomiting.[2,6]

Uterine inversion is more common in primigravidae women.[7,10] Other predisposing factors include:

- fundal position of the placenta[2]

- short umbilical cord

- abnormality of the placenta (e.g. placenta accreta)

- congenital anomalies of the uterus (e.g. bicornuate uterus)[8]

- gravitational weight of an intrauterine mass (e.g. fibroids).[8]

Diagnosis

The clinical presentation and diagnosis of uterine inversion is dependent on the classification of time and severity.

A first degree inversion may be missed as the fundus will not be visible at the introitus or palpable at the cervix and there may be no signs and symptoms. However, an indentation may be palpable at the fundus.

A second degree inversion will be more recognisable. With a third degree inversion, the uterus is not palpable in the abdomen and on vaginal examination the inverted fundus will be felt in the vagina or be visible at the introitus. The placenta may or may not be attached. A second or third degree inversion requires a prompt response.[2]

Signs and symptoms

There are two cardinal signs, those of shock and pain.

Shock

This is sudden, profound and may be disproportionate to the amount of blood loss and degree of inversion. It occurs in response to neurogenic stimuli and hypovolaemia.[1,11]

Bleeding may or may not be present depending on whether the placenta is attached to the uterine wall.

Pain

This is characteristically severe, low abdominal and accompanied by a down-bearing sensation. It is caused by traction on the infundibular pelvic ligaments, round ligaments and the ovaries.[12,13]

In subacute and chronic inversion, the signs and symptoms may be less dramatic and are classically characterised by urinary retention, chronic heavy lochia and a low pelvic 'dragging' sensation.[13]

Management

Management of acute second and third degree inversion in both hospital and home settings is discussed below.

Evidence and research based protocols for the management of the third stage of labour should be in place in all units. All midwives should be familiar with both the active and expectant management of the third stage of labour. Prophylaxis is crucial to minimise the risk of inversion caused by any mismanagement of the third stage of labour.

Differential diagnoses

As shock is a cardinal sign, it is necessary to exclude a differential diagnosis of pulmonary or amniotic fluid embolism, myocardial infarction and uterine rupture. A prompt vaginal examination will confirm the presence of a uterine inversion and it is important to act quickly to minimise maternal morbidity and mortality. If treatment is delayed the uterus can become oedematous and congested. Delay also allows the formation of a cervical contraction ring, which will impede replacement of the inverted fundus.

Immediate management in hospital

Assistance

As with all acute obstetric emergencies, help must be summoned. This should include a senior obstetrician and an obstetric anaesthetist.

Resuscitation and treatment of shock

The assisting midwife may undertake this while the midwife conducting the delivery attempts to replace the uterus. Once systemic stability has been achieved, the aim of management is to replace the uterus as soon as possible. This needs to be done before the development of a cervical contraction ring. *See* Chapter 2 for treatment and management of shock.

Replacement of the uterus

Whether the placenta has separated or not, an attempt should be made to return the uterus to the vagina if it has prolapsed outside the introitus. Although it may appear easier to replace a smaller mass, no attempt should be made to manually remove the placenta if it has not separated. Removing the placenta will exacerbate shock and cause haemorrhage[14,15] The attached placenta prevents bleeding because the uterine sinuses are not exposed.

Manual repositioning of the uterus

If the uterine fundus is palpable and/or visible, the uterus should be replaced. The preferred method is Johnson's manoeuvre.[6,8,10] The midwife inserts her hand into the vagina and the fundus is cupped in the palm of the hand. Pressure is exerted back up and along the long axis of the vagina towards the posterior fornix until the uterus is back in the vagina. When feeding the uterus back through the cervix, it is important to reposition the last section of the uterus that inverted first to prevent overlapping tissue at the cervix which would further compound oedema and congestion. This position needs to be held for at least five minutes or until a firm contraction occurs to ensure that the uterus remains in the pelvis. Intravenous oxytocics should then be given to maintain uterine contraction, according to unit protocol. This enables the cervix to reform.

If manual removal of the placenta is necessary, this should be done in theatre under general anaesthetic because of the risk of postpartum haemorrhage.

If manual replacement of the uterus fails, then medical or surgical intervention will be necessary. This can be achieved through the introduction of O'Sullivan's hydrostatic method, although this is very rarely performed in modern obstetrics.[5] Alternatively, tocolytic agents such as ritodrine or salbutamol can be used to relax the cervical contraction ring. Once the ring is relaxed, the uterus can be returned manually. If manual replacement continues to fail, surgical intervention via a laparotomy will be required.

Immediate management at home

Removal of the placenta

No attempt should be made to remove the placenta for reasons stated above.

Assistance

Call obstetric paramedics and arrange for immediate transfer into hospital. Alert the nearest consultant-led maternity unit. Whilst waiting for paramedic assistance carry out the following procedures.

Resuscitation and treatment of shock

See Chapter 2 for the treatment and management of shock.

Replacement of the uterus

If the uterus is prolapsed, an attempt should be made to return it to the vagina to prevent further shock and reduce maternal morbidity. If this is not possible, the uterus can be wrapped in sterile gauze soaked in warm saline or water. The use of a plastic bag may help to retain heat and moisture. This can all be wrapped in a towel to maintain moisture and warmth and possibly delay the onset of shock. The plastic bag may also prevent the towel adhering to the uterus.

Ongoing management

Once the woman has been stabilised and the uterus replaced, reflection is essential. This should result in the following actions and advice.

Documentation

It is important that documentation accurately reflects the course of events and treatment. As with all obstetric emergencies, if notes are written retrospectively it is necessary to record this fact when documenting the date and times of the events.

Debriefing

Early debriefing is essential for the mother and her family. The midwife responsible for the case should be involved in this process.

Debriefing and reflection for the midwife

The midwife should be offered an opportunity to reflect on and discuss the case, in particular the management of the third stage of labour. This may be undertaken with the involvement of the supervisor of midwives.

Management of future pregnancies and labours

Because of the risk of repeat inversion, careful consideration needs to be given to the management of the second and third stages of labour in future pregnancies.[10]

Uterine rupture

A uterine rupture is defined as the separation of the pregnant uterine wall, with or without expulsion of the foetus.[5] It is a very serious complication of labour that can lead to foetal death and contributes to maternal morbidity and mortality. It may also occur during pregnancy, usually after 32 weeks' gestation and particularly in the presence of a classic longitudinal uterine scar.[14]

The incidence of complete spontaneous uterine rupture is rare. However, incomplete rupture or scar dehiscence is 1:200 in the developing world and 1:1500 in the developed world.[2] The rate for the developed world does not seem to be falling because of the increase in caesarean section.

The risk of uterine rupture increases in women who have had a previous caesarean section. There is more risk if the time interval between labour and the previous caesarean section is less than 18 months. Uterine rupture is less common when any scar from a previous caesarean section is in the lower segment because this is the portion of the uterus that does not contract.

The incidence of uterine rupture is greater in women who have had a classic uterine incision as this involves the contractile portion of the uterus. As a consequence initial healing during involution may be disrupted and/or contractions during a subsequent pregnancy and labour may disrupt the scar.

Classification

There are three generally accepted classifications, described below.

A complete (true) rupture involves a full thickness tear of the uterine wall and pelvic peritoneum.[16] Usually all or part of the foetus extrudes into the peritoneal cavity. The complete rupture may involve a previous uterine scar.

An incomplete (silent or occult) rupture involves a tear of the myometrium but not the peritoneum. It is commonly associated with a previous lower segment caesarean section scar.[2,16]

Scar dehiscence involves a thinning or tearing of the uterine wall along an old scar. The foetal membranes remain intact and the foetus is not expelled into the peritoneal cavity.[6,14]

Aetiology

A traumatic uterine rupture can be associated with the following:

- poor management of induction and augmentation of labour, including the misuse of oxytocic drugs especially in the case of a previously scarred uterus[12,14]

- use of oxytocics in an attempt to augment an undiagnosed obstructed labour[2]

- instrumental deliveries, especially high cavity and rotational forceps[2,14]

- manipulation during pregnancy or labour to correct an unstable lie or malpresentation (e.g. external cephalic or internal podalic versions)

- manual removal of the placenta

- shoulder dystocia

- use of fundal pressure in the second stage of labour

- blunt or direct trauma (e.g. motor vehicle accident).

A spontaneous uterine rupture can be associated with the following:

- previous uterine surgery (e.g. classic caesarean section incision or myomectomy)[14]
- strong uterine contraction without the use of oxytocic drugs[2]
- unrecognised previous uterine trauma (e.g. weakening of the uterine wall during curettage)
- obstructed labour leading to tonic uterine action and excessive thinning of lower segment
- placental abruption, due to distension and abruption of the uterine wall.

Other contributory factors to uterine rupture are the implantation of the placenta over the site of a previous uterine scar and multiparity because of progressive fibrosis and thinning of the uterine muscle.[2]

Signs and symptoms

These vary greatly and depend on the stage of labour and degree of rupture or dehiscence.

Complete rupture

- Severe tearing, abdominal pain or persistent lower abdominal pain and tenderness that continues between contractions.
- Maternal shock: the degree is dependent on the extent of the rupture.
- Fresh bleeding from the vagina.
- Foetal heart rate abnormalities (e.g. tachycardia and/or variable and late decelerations).
- Severe foetal distress or intrauterine foetal death.
- Cessation of labour.
- Palpation of the foetus in the abdomen.
- Haematuria, because the bladder is often adherent to a previous uterine scar.

Incomplete rupture

There may be no signs and symptoms. However, if present their onset is gradual.[6]

- Labour may slow down especially in primigravida women.
- May only be diagnosed retrospectively at caesarean section or at laparotomy investigation for postpartum haemorrhage.

The use of epidural pain relief in labour is not thought to mask the pain or tenderness of uterine rupture.[2,17]

Management

Management in hospital

- Stop oxytocin infusion if it is being used.
- Summon help. As with all acute obstetric emergencies this should include a senior obstetrician and an obstetric anaesthetist.
- Resuscitate and treat the shock (*see* Chapter 2 for treatment and management of shock).
- Obtain consents and prepare for surgical delivery or laparotomy.

Management at home

Early recognition of signs and symptoms is essential.

- Summon help. Call obstetric paramedics and arrange for immediate transfer into hospital. Alert the nearest consultant-led maternity unit.
- Resuscitate and treat shock whilst waiting for paramedic assistance (*see* Chapter 2).

Conclusion

As women with pre-existing uterine scars are the group most at risk of uterine rupture, careful consideration must be given when planning the management of future pregnancies and labours. However, the long held guiding principle of 'once a caesarean, always a caesarean' is no longer the accepted mantra in most maternity units.

Induction of labour (IOL) for women with previous caesarean scars is a controversial issue. The Royal College of Obstetricians and Gynaecologists (RCOG) guidelines[18] from which the National Institute for Clinical Excellence clinical guidelines[19] are derived comment on the rarity of randomised controlled trials (RCT) on this group of women. Only four RCTs have been published and these included a total of only 137 women. This provides insufficient data to evaluate the risks of IOL on such women. Therefore it was difficult for the RCOG to make recommendations for practice.

Adherence to safe guiding principles should allow the majority of women who choose vaginal birth after a previous caesarean to deliver with minimal risk.[2] However, these women should be carefully selected. Information about the previous caesarean section, including pre-operative events and postoperative recovery, should be carefully scrutinised. The RCOG recommends that the women's views and wishes should be borne in mind when making plans for delivery.[18]

For women with previous caesarean section scars, limited use of prostaglandin pessaries for IOL appears to be safe.[2] However, if the cervix is very unfavourable and remains so after the second attempt at induction, using small amounts of prostaglandin each time, indications for IOL and further management should be reassessed. Extreme caution is advocated when considering using oxytocin for augmentation.

Labour and vaginal delivery following previous caesarean section can therefore be recommended providing the following points apply.

- There has been early counselling and education on the signs and symptoms of uterine scar separation. This will facilitate an informed decision and choice on the part of the pregnant woman with regard to the place and mode of delivery.

- Sufficient obstetric and anaesthetic backup is readily available in the maternity unit.

- Women with risk factors have been identified. This group should have an agreed, documented plan of management for labour and delivery. This should include a readiness to proceed to emergency caesarean section in the event of prolonged labour, foetal distress or scar pain, any or all of which may indicate imminent scar dehiscence or uterine rupture.

References

1 Moretti ML and Sibai BM (1990) Peripartum emergencies. In: GI Benrubi (ed) *Obstetric Emergencies.* Churchill Livingstone, New York.

2 Baskett TF (1999) *Essential Management of Obstetric Emergencies* (3e). Clinical Press, Bristol.

3 Cavanagh D and Roa P (1982) Uterine inversion. In: D Cavanagh, RE Wood, TCF O'Conner and RA Knupple (eds) *Obstetric Emergencies* (3e). Harper and Row, Cambridge.

4 Nel JT (1995) *Core Obstetrics and Gynaecology.* Butterworth, South Africa.

5 Park EH and Sachs BP (1999) Postpartum hemorrhage and other problems of the third stage. In: DK James, PJ Steer, CP Weiner and B Gonik (eds) *High Risk Pregnancy Management Options* (2e). WB Saunders, London.

6 Shiers C (1999) Midwifery and obstetric emergencies. In: VR Bennett and LK Brown (eds) *Myles Textbook for Midwives* (13e). Churchill Livingstone, Edinburgh.

7 Brar HS, Greenspoon JS, Platt LD and Paull RH (1989) Acute puerperal inversion. *J Repro Med.* **34** (2): 173–7.

8 Irani S and Jordan J (1997) Management of uterine inversion. *Curr Obstet Gynaecol.* **7**: 232–5.

9 Benedetti T (2001) Obstetric haemorrhage. In: SG Gabbe, JR Niebyl and JL Simpson (eds) *Obstetrics: normal and problem pregnancies* (4e). Churchill Livingstone, New York.

10 Watson P, Besch N and Bowes WA (1980) Management of acute and sub acute puerperal inversion of the uterus. *Obstet Gynecol.* **55** (1): 12.

11 Chamberlain G (ed) (1995) *Obstetrics by Ten Teachers* (16e). Edward Arnold, London.

12 Pearce JM and Steele SA (1987) *A Manual of Labour Ward Practice.* John Wiley, London.

13 Kean LH (2000) Other problems of the third stage. In: LH Kean, PN Baker and DI Edelstone (eds) *Best Practice in Labour Ward Management* (1e). WB Saunders, Edinburgh.

14 Cunningham FG, McDonald PC, Gant NF, Leveno KJ and Gilstrap LC (1997) Obstetric hemorrhage. In: JW Williams (ed) *Williams Obstetrics* (19e). Prentice Hall, London.

15 Jyothi NK, Cox C and Johanson R (2001) Management of obstetric emergencies and trauma (MOET): regional questionnaire survey of obstetric practice among career obstetricians in the UK. *J Obst Gynaecol.* **21** (2): 107–11.

16 Cavanagh D and Wood RE (1982) Haemorrhage. In: D Cavanagh, RE Wood, TCF O'Conner and RA Knupple (eds) *Obstetric Emergencies* (3e). Harper and Row, Cambridge.

17 Miller AWF and Hanretty KP (1997) *Obstetrics illustrated* (5e). Churchill Livingstone, New York.

18 RCOG (2001) *Induction of Labour* (Guideline 9). RCOG Press, London.

19 National Institute for Clinical Excellence (2001) *Inherited Clinical Guideline D: induction of labour*. NICE, London.

CHAPTER 9

Shoulder dystocia and umbilical cord prolapse

Caroline Squire

Shoulder dystocia

'... sometimes the head is so small, and the shoulders so large, that without a very great difficulty they cannot pass, which makes the child remain often in the passage after the head is born ... When the chirurgeon (surgeon) meets with this case, he must speedily deliver the child out of the prison, for a small delay may there strangle the child'.[1] (1697)

Clearly shoulder dystocia as an obstetric emergency has always existed and it is essential that midwives are fully up to date in their knowledge of what to do when it occurs. Optimal maternal and foetal outcomes are possible if the care providers understand the nature of the problem and the mechanisms involved, have a well-defined management plan and are able to function without undue haste or the use of excessive physical force.[2] However, Neill and Sriemevan[3] sent out a questionnaire to 166 midwives and obstetric junior doctors to assess their knowledge of the management of shoulder dystocia and to establish whether mandatory teaching and updating was required. Of the respondents, 58% claimed they were confident in the management of shoulder dystocia, but only 4% gained full marks on the scoring system devised to assess their knowledge. Shoulder dystocia was found to be a major cause of mortality in infants of 4 kg and over in the report of the *Confidential Enquiry into Stillbirths and Deaths in Infancy*.[4]

Definition

There are several definitions of shoulder dystocia to be found in the literature and it may be that practitioners use the term in a general sense to describe a range of difficulties encountered with the delivery of the shoulders (*see* Figure 9.1).[5] This lack of consensus has led to variations in the reported incidence of shoulder dystocia and a possible under reporting of the condition.[6] Furthermore, this lack of consensus has also prevented a true evaluation of the effectiveness of different manoeuvres used in the management of the condition.[7]

One simple definition is that shoulder dystocia occurs when the shoulders fail to traverse the pelvis spontaneously after delivery of the head.[2] Gibb[6] however describes three degrees of shoulder dystocia in order of severity as follows:

- a tight squeeze of a big baby with the normal mechanism of rotation present

- unilateral dystocia where the posterior shoulder has entered the pelvis but the anterior is stuck above the symphysis pubis

- bilateral dystocia where both shoulders are arrested above the pelvic brim.

With the second two types, downward traction will only further impact the shoulders.[8]

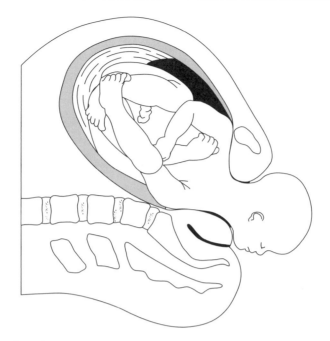

Figure 9.1 Shoulder dystocia

Incidence

The incidence of shoulder dystocia is difficult to calculate given the problems in defining it and that the broader the definition, the higher the recorded incidence. However, a range of between 0.23–2.09% of all vaginal births has been reported, with an increase in risk as the birth weight increases.[9,10] Olugbile and Mascarenhas[11] reviewed shoulder dystocia at the Birmingham Women's Hospital and the rate of incidence they reported was 0.53%.

Prediction and risk factors

Many authors agree that shoulder dystocia often occurs unexpectedly and the first hint of an impending problem may be slow extension of the foetal head. The chin will remain tight against the mother's perineum and the head may look as though it is trying to return into the vagina ('turtle sign').[12–17]

Possible risk factors during the preconception period have been identified by O'Leary[2] (*see* Box 9.1).

Glynn and Olah[18] have identified that the most important antenatal risk factor is a big baby or a previous history of one (*see* Box 9.2).

Box 9.1: Preconception risk factors for shoulder dystocia

- Macrosomic maternal birth weight.
- Prior birth with shoulder dystocia.
- Prior macrosomic infant.
- Glucose excess states (pre-existing diabetes or obesity).
- Multiparity.
- Prior gestational diabetes.
- Advanced maternal age.

Cohen et al.[19] found that in their study of diabetic patients there was a direct correlation between the level of foetal truncal asymmetry measured sonographically and the incidence and severity of shoulder dystocia. However, Lewis et al.[17] found that in their study of data from 1622 women the factors in both the control group and the group of women who experienced shoulder dystocia during their births were not significantly different and included obesity, multiparity, a history of diabetes, short maternal stature, post-maturity and advanced maternal age. Similarly, Blickstein et al.[15] found that shoulder dystocia could not be attributed to any particular difference between the current and previous heaviest birth weight. Even in macrosomic infants, they found that shoulder dystocia and brachial plexus injury are unpredictable. In France, Verspyck et al.[13] attempted to relate maternal and infant characteristics to the shoulder width of the newborn and to evaluate the predictive value of the shoulder width measurement in cases of shoulder dystocia. They found that although the newborn shoulder width measurement correlated strongly with birth weight, it remained a poor predictor for shoulder dystocia. The conclusion must be that clear prediction and identification of risk factors in the antenatal period remain elusive.

Glynn and Olah[18] have identified the following possible intrapartum risk factors (*see* Box 9.3).

It may be that a combination of risk factors multiply the likelihood of shoulder dystocia and can be predictive in individual cases but identification remains easier with the benefit of hindsight.[8]

Potential maternal outcomes

Bowes[20] has identified potential maternal trauma (*see* Box 9.4).

It has been reported that shoulder dystocia associated with fundal pressure leading to uterine rupture and catastrophic haemorrhage has resulted in maternal death.[21] Importantly, it is likely that the mother and her partner may be emotionally traumatised from their experience and may develop post traumatic stress disorder even if the infant survives in reasonable health.[22] It may be useful for a midwife to visit them at home, if they wish, to listen to their experiences. Clearly, subsequent births may also be terrifying for the woman and partner and in these situations midwives need to be especially insightful and sensitive.

Potential foetal outcomes

Possible trauma to the newborn include the following (*see* Box 9.5).[23]

Clavicular fractures are among the most common injuries associated with shoulder dystocia but they also frequently occur in infants weighing

---

Box 9.5: Potential foetal outcomes

- Brachial plexus injury.

- Phrenic nerve injury.

- Fractures of the clavicle or humerus.

- Neonatal asphyxia.

- Death.

---

less than 4000 g.[23] In terms of neurological damage, Erb's palsy is the result of trauma to the fifth and sixth cervical nerves and manifests with absent biceps and Moro reflex on the affected side. Clinically, there is internal rotation and adduction of the shoulder, an unequal Moro reflex, extension and pronation of the elbow and weak wrist extension or the 'waiter's tip' position.[24] Klumpke's palsy concerns the lower trunk lesion at the eighth cervical and first thoracic vertebrae, generally affecting the intrinsic muscles of the hand leading to a claw hand which cannot be closed to make a fist. Horner's syndrome may be present on the affected side due to the involvement of the sympathetic fibres that cross the first thoracic vertebra.[25] Rarely, a severe injury will involve the entire plexus and cause complete paralysis of the arm. Another rare injury concerns the fourth cervical root, which involves trauma to the phrenic nerve and would present with features of respiratory distress with paralysed hemidiaphragm.[23]

The highest risk of fractures and neurological damage occurs when traction and fundal pressure are used together to expedite delivery.[26,27] Midwives need to know that fundal pressure must not be used to relieve shoulder dystocia and experts will testify it is a substandard practice in a court of law.[28] McRoberts' manoeuvre, delivery of the posterior arm and corkscrew manoeuvres are associated with the least trauma for both the mother and the infant.[21,29] However, it has been postulated that brachial plexus injury may occur regardless of the procedure used to disimpact the shoulder.[30,31] Gherman[32] suggests that brachial plexus palsy and bone fracture may arise as a result of the labour process itself or as an intra-uterine event. Brachial plexus injury has been seen to occur after uncomplicated vaginal births, in infants in cephalic presentation during caesarean

section and from the posterior shoulder lodging on the sacral promontory.[32–36] Gonik et al.[35] suggest that spontaneous endogenous forces may contribute substantially to neonatal brachial plexus injury and it may be that stopping pushing until the anterior shoulder is freed will limit injury. Nocon[23] concurs, stating that before the midwife or obstetrician is even aware that shoulder dystocia will occur, the brachial plexus may be significantly stretched due to gentle downward traction exerted to assist the birth of the anterior shoulder and the expulsive efforts of the mother driving the anterior shoulder forward and upward above the symphysis.

Hope et al.[12] reviewed the notes of 56 cases of deaths from shoulder dystocia reported to the *Confidential Enquiry into Stillbirths and Deaths in Infancy*. They found that maternal obesity and big babies were over-represented in pregnancies complicated by fatal shoulder dystocia. The median time interval between delivery of the head and the rest of the body was only five minutes. This is a very short time interval and they postulated that the reasons for cerebral injury and death in shoulder dystocia may be different to those for cerebral hypoxia-ischaemia from other causes such as cord prolapse or placental abruption. They also suggested that long labour, probably causing metabolic acidosis, compression of the neck resulting in cerebral venous obstruction, excessive vagal stimulation and bradycardia, or other mechanisms, may combine with reduced arterial oxygen supply to cause clinical deterioration out of proportion to the duration of hypoxia. There was evidence from some autopsies that trauma as well as hypoxia-ischaemia may have contributed to the adverse outcome. Other mechanisms such as massive vagal stimulation would not be detectable at autopsy.

Importantly, Hope et al.[12] found that the midwife was the lead professional at 65% of these births and middle grade or senior obstetric staff were supervising only 47% of the births by the time the body was delivered. Furthermore, they suggest that the delayed arrival of paediatric staff in many cases was less than beneficial, even if there was no guarantee that earlier paediatric intervention would have altered the outcome. Poor communication between parents and professionals was found in several of these cases and they felt that greater involvement of mothers in antenatal and intrapartum decisions may have helped in some cases.

Avoidance of shoulder dystocia

There are three ways to try to reduce the incidence of shoulder dystocia.[15] The first is to deliver all macrosomic foetuses by caesarean section. Indeed, Gross et al.[37] maintained that elective caesarean delivery may be indicated for infants weighing more that 4500 g. However, although this would obviate the trauma described above to the mother and foetus this suggestion could be criticised because it is difficult to predict macrosomic infants even with the use of ultrasound.[8,14,23,38] Studies have shown that there was a marked increase in caesarean section for babies with a heavy birth weight predicted before delivery but with no significant difference in the incidence of shoulder dystocia or birth trauma.[39,40] Data collected by Blickstein et al.[15] suggest that birth weights of more that 4200 g carry a risk of 1:8–9 for shoulder dystocia and 1:79 for brachial plexus injury. The dilemma is whether to perform unnecessary caesarean sections to avoid these complications given the problems and risks that major abdominal surgery incurs.

The second way to try to reduce the incidence of shoulder dystocia is to avoid macrosomia by inducing suspected cases. However, it seems clear that induction of labour and ripening of a relatively unripe cervix contributes to an excessive caesarean delivery rate with its comcomitant hazards. There is also a risk of iatrogenic prematurity, especially in the early delivery of the diabetic mother. In addition there is the problem of accurate estimation of foetal weight by ultrasound given its wide margin of error at term.[23,41,42] However, it may be that the obstetrician should make a clinical evaluation and opt for induction if the cervix is ripe and the woman is at term.[23]

The third way to attempt to reduce the incidence of shoulder dystocia is to identify any antenatal indicators for the complication (*see* Boxes 9.1 and 9.2). This may raise questions such as whether babies of diabetic mothers be delivered by caesarean section. Although a policy of elective caesarean delivery may be more justifiable in this population, it is still controversial. Nesbitt et al.[38] found that the risk of shoulder dystocia for unassisted and assisted births to diabetic mothers increased as the birth weight increased. Langer et al.[43] considered that elective caesarean delivery for diabetic women with foetuses estimated to weigh more than 4250 g would prevent 76% of shoulder dystocias. However, the findings could be criticised given the difficulty of predicting birth weight of foetuses at term. Conversely, Keller et al.[44] could not justify elective caesarean delivery in gestational diabetic women with foetuses estimated to weigh more than 4000 g because over half of the shoulder dystocias in this group occurred in foetuses that weighed less than 4000 g.

Management at birth

Diagnosis

Timely recognition and accurate management of shoulder dystocia are imperative in preventing birth trauma to the mother and foetus (*see* Box 9.3 for risk factors). The foetal head is born, typically after a long period of bearing down by the exhausted mother, and retracts or recoils against the maternal perineum and then fails to restitute in line with the shoulders. The retraction of the foetal head is known as the 'turtle sign'.[20] Even if external rotation is accomplished, lateral traction of normal force is ineffective in delivering the anterior shoulder beneath the symphysis. Forceful lateral traction should be avoided as this is likely to cause greater impaction of the shoulders against the pelvic inlet.[45] If shoulder dystocia occurs at a home birth, the ambulance should be summoned and transfer to hospital should be as swift as possible in order to gain access to neonatal resuscitation facilities. The maternity unit should be informed of what is happening prior to arrival. A situation such as this serves to emphasise the importance of having two midwives present at home births so that one can make the necessary telephone calls to summon assistance and both can help the other in terms of clinical decision-making and giving emotional support.

Manoeuvres to expedite delivery

The various manoeuvres are described below. It is important to realise, however, that no single manoeuvre has been proven to be superior to any other in disimpacting the shoulder and none is entirely free from potential injury to the foetus or mother.[23] Nocon[23] found that regardless of the manoeuvre used, about 15–20% of infants suffer some injury, albeit transitory. He feels that no protocol should serve as a substitute for clinical judgement because there is no rationale for choosing one technique over another.

Box 9.6: Drill for shoulder dystocia

H Help! Call for help; activate protocol.

E Episiotomy: enables better access to the foetus and for internal manoeuvres.

L Legs: McRoberts' manoeuvre (30–60 seconds).

P Pressure: external suprapubic (30–60 seconds).

E Enter the vagina: Wood's screw; Rubin's (30–60 seconds).

R Remove the posterior arm.

R Roll over onto all fours.

Z Zavanelli manoeuvre: included here although not strictly part of the mnemonic.

Although shoulder dystocia is rare it creates an urgent situation, so there should be regular multi-disciplinary review and reflection on manoeuvres. A mnemonic designed to help midwives and other clinicians involved with births complicated with shoulder dystocia is described in Box 9.6.[46]

Disimpaction manoeuvres

The McRoberts' manoeuvre

This manoeuvre involves hyperflexion of the woman's legs into a knee–chest position and is simple to apply (*see* Figure 9.2). It has been associated with lower levels of maternal and foetal morbidity.[29] When used alone, McRoberts' manoeuvre has alleviated approximately 40% of all shoulder dystocia cases and this rises to 54% when it is combined with suprapubic pressure. Furthermore, its use can reduce foetal shoulder extraction force and brachial plexus stretching which may help reduce the incidence of palsy due to brachial plexus damage.[47] Gherman et al.[48] analysed the McRoberts' manoeuvre by x-ray pelvimetry and found that it does not change the actual dimension of the maternal pelvis, but that it does straighten the sacrum relative to the lumbar spine and may enable the symphysis pubis to rotate superiorly and slide over the foetal shoulder. It also reduces the angle of inclination. Smeltzer[49] considers that the McRoberts' manoeuvre elevates

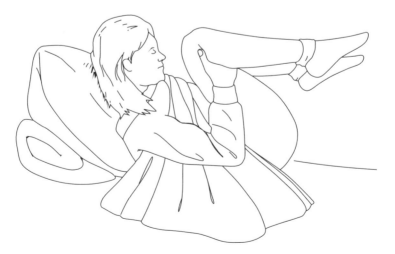

Figure 9.2 McRoberts' manoeuvre

the anterior foetal shoulder and flexes the foetal spine. The action of lifting and flexion pushes the posterior shoulder over the sacrum and through the pelvic inlet and straightens the maternal spine. Also, the superior rotation of the symphysis pubis will bring the plane of the pelvic inlet perpendicular to the maximum maternal expulsive force.[50] Although the woman may be able to hyperflex her hips herself, if she has had an epidural it may be necessary for the midwife to ask for two assistants, one for each leg.[51]

The McRoberts' manoeuvre is recommended as the initial technique in the management of shoulder dystocia because it does not involve manipulation of the foetus and would seem to be relatively safe. However, Gherman et al. published a case study[52] in which it seemed that symphysis separation and transient femoral neuropathy were associated with this manoeuvre. They postulate that an overly exaggerated lithotomy position and thigh abduction stretches the articular surfaces of the symphysis pubis and that increased pressure is placed on the femoral nerve by the overlying inguinal ligament.

Suprapubic pressure

Suprapubic pressure is another non-invasive disimpaction manoeuvre and should be considered as a second step because its use may result in clavicular fractures.[53] Before suprapubic pressure is attempted, the maternal bladder should be empty to avoid bladder trauma and impediment to shoulder rotation. The method advocated is to apply gentle pressure with the palm or the heel

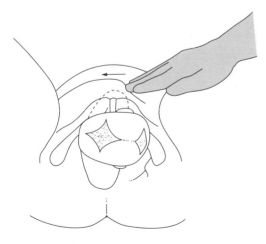

Figure 9.3 Suprapubic pressure

of the hand against the foetal back, directing the pressure towards the foetal midline (*see* Figure 9.3). This will adduct the shoulders and may decrease the bisacromial diameter allowing the shoulder to rotate off the pubic bone and into the pelvis. Usually, this procedure is used in conjunction with other manoeuvres, commonly the McRoberts' manoeuvre. Clearly, it is important to know the position of the foetus beforehand otherwise the bisacromial diameter will increase and cause the situation to become even more serious.

All-fours manoeuvre

If the McRoberts' manoeuvre is not the most appropriate initial response to suspected shoulder dystocia, then women and midwives may find the all-fours position useful. The actual movement of the woman turning onto her hands and knees may help dislodge the shoulder, particularly if it is the posterior shoulder that is impacted behind the sacral promontory, although the anterior shoulder could remain wedged against the symphysis pubis. Furthermore, the midwife loses eye contact with the mother which may make communication at this crucial time more difficult.[50] However, Bruner et al.[54] felt that the all-fours manoeuvre appeared to be a rapid, safe and effective technique for reducing shoulder dystocia in labouring women. They were enthusiastic in their appraisal of the manoeuvre and make it clear that the all-fours position does not preclude the performance of the other manoeuvres such as the McRoberts' manoeuvre, suprapubic pressure, shoulder rotation, delivery of the posterior arm and even cephalic replacement.

Rotation manoeuvres and manoeuvres involving manipulation of the foetus

Woods' screw rotational manoeuvre

This involves an assistant exerting gentle downward pressure on the foetal buttocks with one hand while the midwife places two fingers into the vagina against the anterior chest wall opposite the posterior shoulder and pushes the posterior shoulder backwards through a 180 degree arc (*see* Figure 9.4). As the posterior shoulder rotates, it may deliver or it may free the anterior shoulder for delivery. However, this manoeuvre may result in the abduction of the shoulders which increases

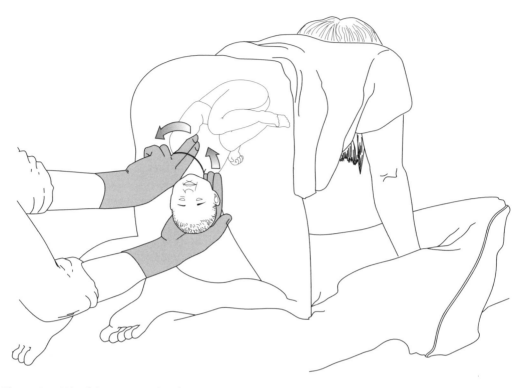

Figure 9.4 Woods' screw rotational manoeuvre

the bisacromial diameter and complicates the problem. For this reason, suprapubic pressure may be applied concurrently to keep the anterior shoulder adducted.[9]

The Rubin manoeuvre

The aim of this manoeuvre is to reduce the bisacromial diameter by adducting the foetal shoulders and it involves the midwife inserting two fingers into the mother's vagina onto the posterior shoulder of the foetus (*see* Figure 9.5). The posterior shoulder may then be displaced by the application of pressure in the direction of the foetal chest.[50] This manoeuvre may be more effective than the Woods' screw manoeuvre because it keeps the shoulders in a forward position or adducted, reducing the bisacromial diameter. Suprapubic pressure may also be applied here so that the anterior shoulder is rocked by pushing from side to side on the mother's abdomen.[53] This may free the anterior shoulder and give the posterior shoulder room to turn.[50]

A variation of the Rubin manoeuvre has also been described as the reverse Woods' screw

manoeuvre by Hall.[53] Several fingers are placed into the vagina against the surface of the scapula of the anterior shoulder which is then rotated forward through a 180 degree arc (*see* Figure 9.6). If the posterior shoulder is more accessible, it may be rotated anteriorly. Whichever shoulder is manoeuvred, the principle is the same so that the shoulders are adducted in order to reduce the bisacromial diameter.

Delivery of the posterior arm

Delivery of the posterior arm is attempted when rotational manoeuvres fail to relieve the impaction of the foetus which is tightly wedged into the pelvic brim. The midwife places two fingers into the vagina under the posterior shoulder and follows the humerus to the elbow (*see* Figure 9.7). Pressure into the antecubital fossa will help the forearm to flex so that it can be swept over the chest. Delivery of the arm may facilitate rotation of the foetus through a 180 degree arc, bringing the posterior shoulder under the symphysis pubis and allowing the rest of the birth to be completed normally.[50,53] Trauma, such as fracture of the

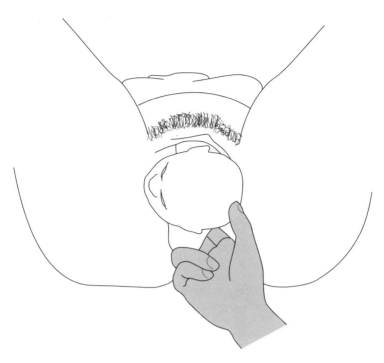

Figure 9.5 Rubin manoeuvre

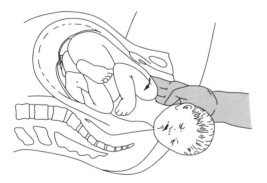

Figure 9.6 Reverse Woods' screw manoeuvre

humerus or clavicle, may occur if the arm is tightly wedged but this may be considered comparatively unimportant at this stage.[8]

Surgical procedures

Episiotomy

An episiotomy is usually performed in order to give extra space at the introitus for the clinician to attempt any direct manoeuvres or manipulation of the foetus. It may be that damage to the perineum is lessened in the long term.

Symphysiotomy

This is the surgical division of the fibrocartilage junction of the symphysis pubis to enlarge the bony pelvis and has been practised for many years in areas of the world where caesarean section is difficult to perform. The procedure is not widely practised in the UK or the USA, possibly due to operator inexperience and maternal morbidity.[55,56] Three case studies were published concerning the use of this procedure. In all cases the infants died, although it should be remembered that all the standard manoeuvres including cephalic replacement had already been performed to no avail and symphysiotomy was performed *in extremis*. Maternal morbidity, including urinary incontinence, was significant but responded to treatment.[55]

Cephalic replacement: Zavanelli manoeuvre

This involves replacing the foetal head into the pelvis for extraction by caesarean section. The head

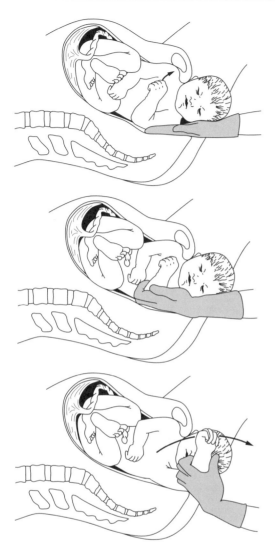

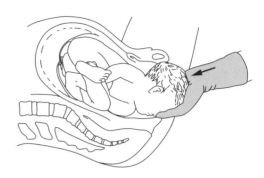

Figure 9.8 Zavanelli manoeuvre

Figure 9.7 Delivery of the posterior arm

five women underwent elective caesarean birth, including four of the five diabetic mothers. Four women had emergency caesarean sections in labour for foetal hypoxia, placental abruption and failure to progress. Of the 42 women delivering vaginally, five experienced a repeated episode of shoulder dystocia. There were no episodes of foetal death or trauma. This gave a repeat recurrence of 9.8% as compared with the total population incidence of 0.58%. The best way to manage subsequent births following one complicated with shoulder dystocia remains unclear. Certainly, the wishes of the mother are as central as are the clinical picture and the judgement of health professionals at the time.

Checklist for midwives

- Enact the HELPERR mnemonic (*see* Box 9.6).
- Remember record-keeping.
- Communicate with the mother and her birth partner. Help her/them debrief later if appropriate.
- Practise the manoeuvres.
- Reflect on your experiences with peers and/or supervisor of midwives.
- Consider risk management issues.

Umbilical cord prolapse

Cord prolapse is defined as prolapse of the umbilical cord alongside (occult) or past the presenting part in the presence of ruptured membranes (*see* Figure 9.9).[64] Cord presentation occurs without the presence of ruptured membranes.

is rotated to a direct occipito-anterior or occipito-posterior position and flexed. Then pressure is applied to the vertex to push the head upwards.[57,58] Various case studies have been published concerning this manoeuvre but at the present time, although it is thought that it should be on every obstetrician's list, it must remain a low priority until its applicability has been demonstrated more clearly.[59–62]

Delivery in subsequent pregnancies

Smith[63] studied 51 case notes of women who had experienced previous births complicated by shoulder dystocia. In the subsequent pregnancy,

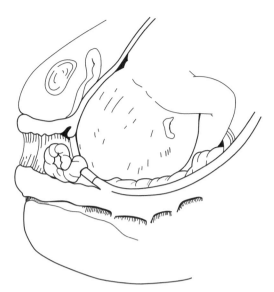

Figure 9.9 Umbilical cord prolapse

Cord prolapse is an obstetric emergency with a reported incidence varying between 1:239 and 1:865 births.[65,66] Reported perinatal mortality ranges between 8.6% and 49% but the extent to which birth asphyxia alone contributes to these figures has not been defined.[65,66] Murphy and MacKenzie[66] examined the management of cord prolapse and occurrence of morbidity and mortality in a retrospective study of 132 babies born after identification of cord prolapse. They concluded that it occurred at a relatively stable rate irrespective of changes in obstetric practices,[67] and that the foetal outcome was not as poor as might be expected, mortality predominantly being attributable to congenital anomalies and prematurity rather than birth asphyxia.

Risk factors

The principle to remember is that whenever there is room for the cord to slip into the pelvis there is the potential for cord presentation or cord prolapse (*see* Box 9.7).

Diagnosis

Cord presentation

This may be diagnosed on vaginal examination when the cord is felt behind intact membranes. It may also be suspected when the midwife detects abnormalities in the foetal heart rate.

Cord prolapse

Umbilical cord prolapse is diagnosed when the cord can be seen externally or palpated in the vagina or alongside the presenting part by the midwife.[69] It may also be suspected when severe, recurrent variable decelerations or bradycardia occur in the foetal heart rate which does not respond to change in maternal position. Once diagnosed, the objective is to maintain the foetal circulation by preventing cord compression and expedite delivery. If the incident occurs at a home birth, then transfer by ambulance should be as swift as possible and the maternity unit should be notified of what is happening prior to arrival. A situation such as this emphasises the importance of having two midwives present at home births.

Box 9.7: Risk factors for cord presentation or prolapse[68]

- Low gestational age.
- Low birth weight.
- Abnormal presentation with an ill-fitting presenting part in the pelvis (i.e. breech).
- Multiple pregnancy particularly with malpresentation of the second foetus.
- High parity (due to non-engagement of the presenting part when the membranes rupture).
- Presenting part is high in the pelvis.
- Polyhydramnios.

Management

It must be remembered that this emergency situation will frighten the mother and her partner, and midwives need to communicate sensitively and explicitly so that the parents understand the gravity of the situation without losing control. Accurate and concurrent record-keeping is essential as is the recording of the foetal heart until delivery is imminent. The following actions may be appropriate for preventing cord compression.

Cord presentation

In the case of cord presentation diagnosed on vaginal examination, the membranes should be left intact and the mother helped into a position that will relieve cord compression (*see* Figures 9.10 and 9.11).

Cord prolapse

1 Manual elevation of the presenting part above the pelvic inlet to relieve cord compression. This is accomplished by the midwife inserting two fingers onto the presenting part and applying pressure.

2 An all-fours position, with buttocks raised and with manual elevation of the presenting part above the pelvic brim (*see* Figure 9.10) or ex-aggerated Sims' position to elevate the woman's buttocks and relieve pressure on the umbilical cord (*see* Figure 9.11). The latter is the more appropriate position for transfer by ambulance.

3 Manual replacement of the umbilical cord (funic reduction) into the vagina.[70] Care must be taken not to handle the cord too much, to prevent spasm of the vessels.

4 Fill the maternal bladder with 400–700 ml of saline solution. This may relieve cord compression and also inhibit uterine contractions, thus decreasing pressure on the cord.[64,68,71]

5 Amnioinfusion of saline or Ringers lactate solution has been described but is not common practice.[72]

If the cervix is fully dilated and the presenting part is engaged, vaginal delivery may be appropriate through maternal effort or with ventouse or forceps. If vaginal delivery is not possible, emergency caesarean section should be performed as soon as possible with prior emptying of the maternal bladder.[64,73,74]

Once the diagnosis of umbilical cord prolapse is made, rapid delivery of the baby is vital. However, in a retrospective review of 65 cases of umbilical cord prolapse it was postulated that the cases of neonatal asphyxia associated with cord prolapse may have been aggravated by factors other than time.[75] It was speculated that the degree of cord compression and the amount of amniotic fluid could affect neonatal outcome. It may be that time spent resuscitating the foetus *in utero* by maternal position changes, inserting a urinary catheter and filling the bladder or administering tocolysis may be beneficial to the foetus and lead to a lower incidence of neonatal asphyxia. The study also found that occult cord

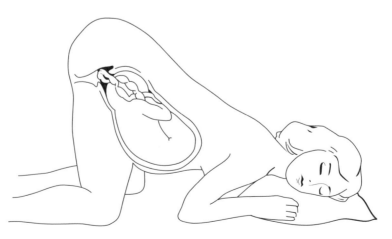

Figure 9.10 All-fours position with buttocks raised

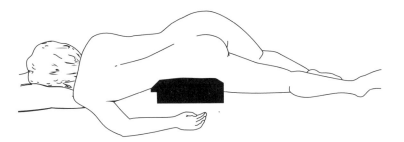

Figure 9.11 Exaggerated Sims' position

prolapse was associated with less perinatal morbidity when compared to frank prolapse.[75]

Checklist for midwives

- Call for help.
- Communicate with the woman and birth partner.
- Relieve cord compression to enable foetal oxygenation: replace cord; maternal position (all fours, buttocks raised or exaggerated Sims'); relieve pressure digitally from the umbilical cord.
- Record-keeping.
- Reflect on experience with peers and/or supervisor of midwives.
- Consider risk management issues.
- Help parents debrief if appropriate.

References

1 Chamberlen H (1697) *The Diseases of Women with Child, and in Child-bed* (3e). Andrew Bell, London.
2 O'Leary JA (1992) *Shoulder dystocia and birth injury.* McGraw-Hill, New York.
3 Neill AM and Sriemevan A (1999) Shoulder Dystocia: room for improvement? *J Obstet Gynaecol.* **19** (2): 132–4.
4 Maternal and Child Health Research Consortium (1997) *Confidential Enquiry into Stillbirths and Deaths in Infancy* (Fourth Annual Report). CESDI, London.
5 Mortimore VR and McNabb M (1998) A six-year retrospective analysis of shoulder dystocia

and delivery of the shoulders. *Midwif.* **14**: 162–73.
6 Gibb D (1995) Clinical focus: shoulder dystocia: the obstetrics. *Clin Focus.* **1**: 49–54.
7 Maternal and Child Health Research Consortium (1995) *Confidential Enquiry into Stillbirth and Deaths in Infancy* (Second Annual Report). CESDI, London.
8 Johnstone FD and Myerscough PR (1998) Shoulder dystocia. *Br J Obstet Gynaecol.* **105**: 811–15.
9 Naef RW and Martin JN (1995) Emergency management of shoulder dystocia. In: JN Martin (ed) *Intrapartum and Postpartum Obstetric Emergencies.* WB Saunders, Philadelphia.
10 Bahar AM (1996) Risk factors and fetal outcome in cases of shoulder dystocia compared with normal deliveries of a similar birth weight. *Br J Obstet Gynaecol.* **103**: 868–72.
11 Olugbile A and Mascarenhas L (2000) Review of shoulder dystocia at the Birmingham Women's Hospital. *J Obstet Gynaecol.* **20** (3): 267–70.
12 Hope P, Breslin S, Lamont L et al. (1998) Fatal shoulder dystocia: a review of 56 cases reported to the confidential enquiry into stillbirths and deaths in infancy. *Br J Obstet Gynaecol.* **105**: 1256–61.
13 Verspyck E, Goffinet F, Hellow MF et al. (1999) Newborn shoulder width: a prospective study of 2222 consecutive measurements. *Br J Obstet Gynaecol.* **106**: 589–92.
14 Gonen R, Spiegel D and Abend M (1996) Is macrosomia predictable and are shoulder dystocia and birth trauma preventable? *Obstet Gynecol.* **88** (4:1): 526–9.
15 Blickstein I, Ben-Arie A and Hagay ZJ (1998) Antepartum risks of shoulder dystocia and brachial plexus injury for infants weighing

4200 g or more. *Gynecol Obstet Invest.* **45**: 77–80.

16 Coates T (1997) Shoulder dystocia: diagnosis, prediction and risk factors. *Mod Midwife.* **7** (8): 12–14.

17 Lewis DF, Edwards MS, Asrat T et al. (1998) Can shoulder dystocia be predicted? *J Repro Med.* **43** (8): 654–8.

18 Glynn M and Olah KS (1994) The management of shoulder dystocia. *Br J Midwif.* **2** (3): 108–12.

19 Cohen BF, Penning S, Ansley D, Porto M and Garite T (1999) The incidence and severity of shoulder dystocia correlates with a sonographic measurement of asymmetry in patients with diabetes. *Am J Perinatol.* **16** (4): 197–201.

20 Bowes WA (1994) Clinical aspects of normal and abnormal labor: shoulder dystocia. In: RK Creasy and R Resnik (eds) *Maternal-Fetal Medicine: principles and practice* (3e). WB Saunders, Philadelphia.

21 Al-Najashi S, Al-Suleiman SA, El-Yahia A et al. (1989) Shoulder dystocia – a clinical study of 56 cases. *Aus NZ J Obstet Gynecol.* **29**: 129–31.

22 Menage J (1996) Post traumatic stress disorder following obstetric/gynaecological procedures. *Br J Midwif.* 4 (10): 532–3.

23 Nocon JJ (2000) Shoulder dystocia and macrosomia. In: LH Kean, PN Baker and DI Edelstone (eds) *Best Practice in Labor Ward Management.* WB Saunders, London.

24 Ubachs JMH, Slooff ACJ and Peeters LLH (1995) Obstetric antecedents of surgically treated obstetric brachial plexus injuries. *Br J Obstet Gynaecol.* **102**: 813–17.

25 Swaiman KF and Wright FS (1982) *The Practice of Pediatric Neurology* (2e). Mosby, St Louis.

26 Gross SJ, Shime J and Farine D (1987) Shoulder dystocia: predictors and outcome: a five year review. *Am J Obstet Gynecol.* **56** (2): 334–6.

27 Bahar AM (1996) Risk factors and fetal outcome in cases of shoulder dystocia compared with normal deliveries of a similar birthweight. *Br J Obstet Gynaecol.* **103**: 868–72.

28 Tolin J (1992) The attorney's viewpoint. In: JA O'Leary (ed) *Shoulder Dystocia and Birth Injury: prevention and treatment.* McGraw Hill, New York.

29 Gherman RB, Goodwin TM, Souter I et al. (1997) The McRoberts' maneuver for the alleviation of shoulder dystocia: how successful is it? *Am J Obstet Gynecol.* **176** (3): 656–61.

30 Gherman RB, Joseph G, Ouzounian JG and Murphy Goodwin T (1998) Obstetric maneuvers for shoulder dystocia and associated fetal morbidity. *Am J Obstet Gynecol.* **178** (6): 1126–30.

31 McFarland MB, Langer O, Piper JM and Berkus MD (1996) Perinatal outcome and the type and number of maneuvers in shoulder dystocia. *Int J Obstet Gynecol.* **55**: 219–24.

32 Gherman RB, Goodwin TM and Ouzounian JG (1997) Brachial plexus palsy associated with cesarean section: an in utero injury? *Am J Obstet Gynecol.* **177**: 1162–4.

33 Jennett RJ, Tarby TJ and Kreinick CJ (1992) Brachial plexus palsy: an old problem revisited. *Am J Obstet Gynecol.* **166**: 1673–7.

34 Gherman RB, Ouzounian JG, Miller DA et al. (1998) Spontaneous vaginal delivery: a risk factor for Erb's palsy. *Am J Obstet Gynecol.* **178**: 423–7.

35 Gonik B, Walker A and Grimm M (2000) Mathematic modelling of forces associated with shoulder dystocia: a comparison of endogenous and exogenous sources. *Am J Obstet Gynecol.* **182**: 689–91.

36 Hankins GDV and Clark SL (1995) Brachial plexus palsy involving the posterior shoulder at spontaneous vaginal delivery. *Am J Obstet Gynecol.* **12**: 44–5.

37 Gross TL, Sokol RJ, Williams T et al. (1987) Shoulder dystocia: a fetal–physician risk. *Am J Obstet Gynecol.* **156**: 1408–18.

38 Nesbitt TS, Gilbert WM and Herrchen B (1998) Shoulder dystocia and associated risk factors with macrosomic infants born in California. *Am J Obstet Gynecol.* **179**: 476–80.

39 Levine AB, Lockwood CJ, Brown B et al. (1992) Sonographic diagnosis of the large for gestational age fetus at term: does it make a difference? *Obstet Gynecol.* **79**: 55–8.

40 Weeks JW, Pitman T and Spinnato JA (1995) Fetal macrosomia: does antenatal prediction affect delivery route and birth outcome? *Am J Obstet Gynecol.* **173**: 1215–19.

41 Delpapa EH and Mueller-Heubach E (1991) Pregnancy outcome following ultrasound diagnosis of macrosomia. *Obstet Gynecol.* **78**: 340–3.

42 Combs CA, Singh NB and Khoury JC (1993) Elective induction versus spontaneous labor after sonographic diagnosis of fetal macrosomia. *Obstet Gynecol.* **81**: 492–6.

43 Langer O, Berkus M, Huff RW et al. (1991) Shoulder dystocia: should the fetus weighing more than 4000 g be delivered by cesarean section? *Am J Obstet Gynecol.* **165**: 831–7.

44 Keller JD, Lopez-Zeno JA, Dooley SL et al. (1991) Shoulder dystocia and birth trauma in gestational diabetes: a five year experience. *Am J Obstet Gynecol.* **165**: 928–30.

45 Benedetti TJ (1995) Shoulder dystocia. *Contemp Obstet Gynecol.* **40** (3): 39–43.

46 American Academy of Family Physicians (1996) *Advanced Life Support in Obstetrics.* American Academy of Family Physicians, Newcastle upon Tyne.

47 Gonik B, Allen R and Sorab J (1989) Objective evaluation of the shoulder dystocia phenomenon: effect of maternal pelvic orientation on force reduction. *Obstet Gynecol.* **74**: 44–7.

48 Gherman RB, Tramont J, Muffley P et al. (2000) Analysis of McRoberts' maneuver by x-ray pelvimetry. *Obstet Gynecol.* **95** (1): 43–7.

49 Smeltzer JS (1986) Prevention and management of shoulder dystocia. *Clin Obstet Gynecol.* **29** (2): 299–308.

50 Coates T (1997) Manoeuvres for the relief of shoulder dystocia. *Mod Midwife.* **7** (9): 15–19.

51 Naef RW and Morrison JC (1994) Guidelines for management of shoulder dystocia. *J Perinatol.* **14** (6): 435–41.

52 Gherman RB, Ouzounian JG, Incerpi MH et al. (1998) Symphyseal separation and transient femoral neuropathy associated with the McRoberts' maneuver. *Am J Obstet Gynecol.* **178**: 609–10.

53 Hall SP (1997) The nurse's role in the identification of risks and treatment of shoulder dystocia. *J Obstet Gynecol Neonatal Nurs.* **26**: 25–32.

54 Bruner JP, Drummond SB, Meenan AL et al. (1998) All-fours maneuver for reducing shoulder dystocia during labor. *J Repro Med.* **43**: 439–43.

55 Murphy Goodwin T, Banks E, Millar LK et al. (1997) Catastrophic shoulder dystocia and emergency symphysiotomy. *Am J Obstet Gynecol.* **177**: 463–4.

56 Reid PC and Osuagwu FI (1999) Symphysiotomy in shoulder dystocia. *J Obstet Gynaecol.* **19** (6): 664–6.

57 Sandberg EC (1985) The Zavanelli maneuvre: a potentially revolutionary method for the resolution of shoulder dystocia. *Am J Obstet Gynecol.* **152**: 479–84.

58 O'Leary JA (1993) Cephalic replacement for shoulder dystocia: present status and future role of the Zavanelli maneuver. *Obstet Gynecol.* **82**: 847–50.

59 Namis NN (1995) Cephalic replacement (the Zavanelli manoeuvre): a desperate solution for severe shoulder dystocia. *Soc Obstet Gynaecol Can.* **17**: 1017–20.

60 Buist R and Khalid O (1999) Successful Zavanelli manoeuvre for shoulder dystocia with an occipitoposterior position. *Aus NZ J Obstet Gynecol.* **39** (3): 310–11.

61 Sandberg EC (1999) The Zavanelli maneuver: 12 years of recorded experience. *Obstet Gynecol.* **93**: 312–17.

62 Vollebergh JHA and van Dongen PWJ (2000) The Zavanelli manoeuvre in shoulder dystocia: case report and review of published cases. *Eur J Obstet Gynaecol Repro Biol.* **89**: 81–4.

63 Smith RB, Lane C and Pearson JF (1994) Shoulder dystocia: what happens at the next delivery? *Br J Obstet Gynaecol.* **101**: 713–15.

64 Johanson R and Cox C (1999) Cord prolapse. In: C Cox and K Grady (eds) *Managing Obstetric Emergencies.* Bios Scientific Publishers, Oxford.

65 Mesleh R, Sultan M, Sabagh T et al. (1993) Umbilical cord prolapse. *J Obstet Gynaecol.* **13**: 24–8.

66 Murphy DJ and MacKenzie IZ (1995) The mortality and morbidity associated with umbilical cord prolapse. *Br J Obstet Gynaecol.* **102**: 826–30.

67 Roberts WE, Martin RW, Roach HH et al. (1997) Are obstetric interventions such as cervical ripening, induction of labor, amnioinfusion or amniotomy associated with umbilical cord prolapse? *Am J Obstet Gynecol.* **176** (6): 1181–5.

68 McGeown P (2001) Practice recommendations for obstetric emergencies. *Br J Midwif.* **9** (2): 71–3.

69 Griese ME and Prickett SA (1992) Nursing management of umbilical cord prolapse. *J Obstet Gynecol Neonatal Nurs.* **22** (4): 311–15.

70 Barrett JM (1991) Funic reduction for the management of umbilical cord prolapse. *Am J Obstet Gynecol.* **165** (3): 654–7.

71 Runnebaum IB and Katz M (1999) Intra-uterine resuscitation by rapid urinary bladder instillation in a case of occult prolapse of an excessively long umbilical cord. *Eur J Obstet Gynecol Repro Biol.* **84** (1): 101–2.

72 Hofmeyr GJ (2000) Amnioinfusion for umbilical cord compression in labour. In: *The Cochrane Library* (Issue 4). Update Software, Oxford.

73 Usta IM, Mercer BM and Sibai BM (1999) Current obstetrical practice and umbilical cord prolapse. *Am J Perinatol.* **16** (9): 479–84.

74 Critchlow CW, Leet TL, Benedetti TJ and Daling JR (1994) Risk factors and infant outcomes associated with umbilical cord prolapse: a population-based case-control study among births in Washington State. *Am J Obstet Gynecol.* **170**: 613–18.

75 Prabulos A-M and Philipson EH (1998) Umbilical cord prolapse: is the time from diagnosis to delivery critical? *J Repro Med.* **43**: 129–32.

CHAPTER 10

Intrapartum and primary postpartum haemorrhage

Helen Crafter

Introduction

When the usually joyous event of birth is accompanied by excessive bleeding in the mother, the atmosphere in the birth room can change very quickly from being one of calm supportiveness to one of bustling intensity. Yet if the midwife and other health professionals are knowledgeable, well-equipped and confident in their skills, most cases of haemorrhage can be prevented from causing long-term physical damage or emotional trauma to the mother. However, there is no place for complacency. Severe obstetric haemorrhage when it does occur can be lethal and if it does not kill, it can leave women physically damaged and all the family deeply distressed by a traumatic birth event. This chapter aims to equip midwives with the knowledge and confidence to prevent and deal with excessive bleeding at and around the time of birth.

Intrapartum haemorrhage (IPH) and primary postpartum haemorrhage (PPH) are commonly defined as excessive blood loss from the genital tract during labour or in the 24 hours following it respectively, of 500 ml or more, or of any amount that compromises the well-being of the mother. However these definitions are open to challenge. Well-nourished pregnant women may lose significantly more blood than 500 ml with no ill effects and before they notice the light-headedness

which accompanies acute anaemia. Indeed pregnant women may lose up to a third of their blood volume (1500–1800 ml) without showing signs of shock.[1] However, this is hardly surprising given that before pregnancy women have a circulating blood volume of approximately four litres and at term this has risen by an average of 50%, with anything from 20–100% being normal.[2] The definition is perhaps more appropriate to the less well-nourished women of previous decades in the Western world and of women living in poverty today, particularly in poor countries. Yet most health professionals would argue that it is the woman's overall condition that should indicate to her midwife whether or not she has lost an excessive amount of blood and this will be dictated by her haematological status prior to labour and the events that occur during it. Another problem of defining intrapartum and postpartum blood loss by amount is that it is known that estimation of blood loss at delivery by health professionals is highly inaccurate and becomes more inaccurate the more blood a woman loses.[3,4] In addition blood often remains concealed as a retro-placental clot. Finally, a good midwife does not wait for 500 ml of blood to trickle or gush from the vagina at birth before she acts. If she sees the potential for excessive blood loss unfolding, she acts promptly to try to prevent a haemorrhage or reduce the blood loss. The most important part of the definition of IPH and primary PPH above is therefore '… any amount of blood loss that compromises the well-being of the mother'. However, it should always be borne in mind that compromise to the mother's condition may not be apparent until she has lost a dangerous amount of blood.

Thorough knowledge of the physiology of labour, both physiologically occurring and actively managed, is assumed. This chapter concentrates more on contemporaneous evidence about which actions are effective when a woman bleeds excessively.

Incidence of severe obstetric haemorrhage

In a study of nearly 50 000 women who gave birth in the South East Thames region over a 12-month period in 1997–98, Waterstone and colleagues[5] calculated the severe morbidity rate from obstetric haemorrhage to be 6.7 in every 1000 deliveries, out of a total severe obstetric morbidity rate of 12.0 in every 1000 deliveries. In this study severe haemorrhage was defined as an estimated blood loss of more than 1500 ml, a peripartum fall in haemoglobin concentration of 4 g/dl or an immediate blood transfusion of four or more units of blood.

By any standard these figures suggest that obstetric haemorrhage is a condition requiring the utmost respect from health professionals responsible at birth in understanding the underlying pathology and being knowledgeable and skilful in dealing with such an event.

In the last *Report on Confidential Enquiries into Maternal Deaths*[6] seven women in the UK were reported to have died from a cause directly related to haemorrhage. Three of these cases were due to placenta praevia, three to placental abruption and one to PPH.

Causes and predisposing factors

Any combination of the causes (*see* Box 10.1) or predisposing factors (*see* Box 10.2) will increase the risk of IPH and early PPH.

The main causes of IPH and early PPH, other than atonic uterus and vasa praevia are well documented elsewhere (*see* Chapters 5 and 7).

Box 10.1: Causes

- Placental abruption.
- Placenta praevia.
- Ruptured uterus.
- Cervical or vaginal lacerations.
- Atonic uterus.
- Ruptured vasa praevia leading to foetal haemorrhage.

Box 10.2: Predisposing factors

- Raised blood pressure (more than 140/90 mmHg).
- Polyhydramnios or multiple pregnancy.
- Previous caesarean section.
- Prolonged labour.
- Injudicious use of Syntocinon®.
- Precipitate labour.
- Supine or semi-recumbent birth.
- Instrumental delivery.
- Caesarean delivery.
- Mismanagement of the third stage of labour.
- General anaesthesia.
- Clotting disorder.

The predisposing factors also warrant attention because contemporary evidence is increasingly becoming available as to how they affect haemostasis before and after the third stage of labour and how individual conditions should best be managed. Each will be discussed separately here.

Atonic uterus

The uterus literally 'lacks muscle tone' because the myometrium fails to contract and retract as or after the placenta separates. The ruptured blood vessels, common in the normal third stage of labour, at the placental site are not compressed by the living ligature action of the myometrial fibres and bleeding is not controlled. It is worth remembering that in pregnancy at least 500 ml of blood crosses the placenta every minute[7] and so atony can lead to rapid, heavy blood loss if efficient uterine action is not speedily achieved. Uterine atony is most commonly associated with incomplete separation of the placenta, retained cotyledon, membrane or blood clot, precipitate or prolonged labour, placenta praevia or abruption, general anaesthesia or mismanagement of the third stage. Sometimes its aetiology is unknown. Elizabeth Davis,[8] an American midwife and author, suggests that maternal position may be a factor.

Vasa praevia

Vasa praevia is associated with a velamentous insertion of the cord into a low-lying placenta. Foetal blood vessels running through the membranes between the umbilical cord and the placenta lie in the lower segment of the uterus in front of the presenting part of the foetus. When the membranes rupture, a foetal vessel may also rupture giving rise to severe foetal bleeding.

Raised blood pressure

Placental abruption is found to be associated in 40 to 50% of cases with maternal hypertension of more than 140/90 mmHg.[9] Importantly for the management of maternal haemorrhage either before or after the birth, pre-eclampsia can fulminate in as little as two hours, so a woman presenting with a primary diagnosis of acute haemorrhage may have undiagnosed pre-eclampsia. Pre-eclampsia may make her blood pressure soar; haemorrhage may make it plummet. One condition may mask the other so different vital signs must be diligently monitored to effect accurate diagnosis and treatment. For all women presenting in labour with haemorrhage these should include a history of pregnancy and present symptoms, general appearance and condition, pulse, urine analysis and a haematological pre-eclampsia screen (*see* Chapter 4).

Polyhydramnios or multiple pregnancy

When the membranes rupture in labour in cases of polyhydramnios or following the birth of the first baby in a multiple pregnancy, the sudden and large reduction in the uterine cavity may precipitate placental separation. Where the uterus is over-stretched in pregnancy, the muscle cells become less able to contract and retract efficiently in the third stage of labour. The cause of PPH is therefore atonic uterus.

Previous caesarean section

A recent history of increasing caesarean section rates is leading to many questions being asked about the effects on future pregnancy of a uterine scar. In a retrospective study Coulter-Smith and colleagues[10] looked for risk factors that are associated with significant obstetric haemorrhage and discovered that over a six-year period of 34 446 deliveries at one hospital, the overall incidence of PPH was 1:931 deliveries. The study found a greater incidence of haemorrhage in parous women, of whom 71% had had a previous caesarean section. While awaiting further research, both mothers and birth attendants need to be aware of this risk factor. A history of one or more caesarean sections is also a risk factor for placenta praevia and placenta accreta in future pregnancies. Caesarean section should therefore be seen in the context of having risk factors for future pregnancies, not just for the present one.

Prolonged labour

Prolonged labour is characterised by weak and uncoordinated contractions. Dehydration, ketosis and tiredness may play a part and ultimately uterine muscle will become exhausted.[7] The resulting inertia can lead to uterine atony.

Injudicious use of prostaglandin and Syntocinon®

Prostaglandins and the drug Syntocinon® should be used with great caution. Whilst useful in inducing labour, and preventing excessively long labour and reducing the caesarean section rate when used wisely, imprudent use can damage both the mother and the baby.[11,12] The use of both prostaglandins and Syntocinon® have been implicated in some cases of uterine rupture in labour, especially if the uterus has been scarred from previous birth or surgery.[12]

After the birth PPH may occur when a Syntocinon® infusion is stopped as soon as the infant is born and, in the absence of enough naturally produced oxytocin, the relaxed uterine muscle fibres allow excessive passage of blood from the recently separated placental vessels.

Therefore Syntocinon® should be discontinued quickly in labour if its use causes problems. However it should not be discontinued abruptly after the birth of the baby and placenta when uterine muscle relaxation is undesirable.

Precipitate labour

Over-efficiency of the uterus in the first and second stages of labour may lead to failure of retraction of the uterine muscle in the third stage. PPH is the result. Also a speedy passage through the birth canal by the foetus can hinder the gradual and gentle stretching of the tissues, which may lead to lacerations of the cervix, vagina and/or perineum, thereby increasing blood loss.[7]

Supine birth

Elizabeth Davis[8] suggests that if a woman gives birth in an upright position, her abdominal organs will naturally compress her uterus against her pelvic floor. However if she gives birth in a supine or semi-recumbent position, she is not afforded this advantage. This is one of many choices available to the midwife in aiming to prevent maternal haemorrhage from atony occurring.

Instrumental delivery

Some of the factors which predispose to ventouse and forceps delivery will also predispose to PPH, such as multiple pregnancy, previous caesarean section and prolonged labour, thereby multiplying the risk. Instrumental delivery is also probably a risk factor in itself, as the natural rhythm of labour is countered by an unnaturally expedited birth

and the necessity for the uterus to contract and retract immediately. Furthermore, women who have an instrumental delivery will almost invariably have an episiotomy which is likely to increase their blood loss. Instrumental delivery also increases the risk of genital tract lacerations.[13,14]

Caesarean delivery

Caesarean birth is almost inevitably associated with a relatively high blood loss because of the amount of tissue incised to reach the baby. Especially in elective surgery maternal oxytocin levels will be low, thereby increasing the risk of atonic uterus, although intravenous Syntocinon® is routinely given to counteract this. The use of general anaesthesia also increases the possibility of PPH (*see* below).

Mismanagement of the third stage

A full bladder in late labour, 'fundus fiddling' (where a health professional applies frequent, irregular pressure to the uterine fundus usually in order to check for good contractility), overstrong cord traction on an unseparated placenta and an inappropriate combination of techniques which should be either actively managed or physiologically managed at the third stage, all contribute to incidence of PPH. All interfere with the normal rhythmic contractions which are designed to exactly co-ordinate muscle contraction and retraction with placental separation, with or without administration of an oxytocic drug.

General anaesthesia

Some commonly used anaesthetic agents such as halothane may cause uterine muscle relaxation.[15]

Clotting disorder

An idiopathic clotting disorder may be present in the mother during pregnancy and its existence may become apparent during routine blood tests, thereby alerting health professionals to an increased risk of bleeding.

Disseminated intravascular coagulopathy (DIC) is an acute condition that occurs when there is a large area of tissue damage, for instance following placental abruption, as a result of pre-eclampsia or eclampsia or following intrauterine foetal death. DIC is very rare when the foetus is alive.[16] A massive release of thromboplastins from the damaged cells into the bloodstream causes widespread clotting throughout the circulation. Clotting factors are used up. Fibrinolysis is triggered and the production of fibrin degradation products (FDPs) further interferes with the process of normal clotting. When no further clotting can take place, uncontrolled bleeding occurs from any site in the body from where blood can escape.

See Box 10.3 for risk reduction measures that can be taken by the midwife and Box 10.8 for further information about the diagnosis and management of DIC.

Diagnosis and management of intrapartum haemorrhage

Bleeding in the first stage of labour may be due to a show (which can be quite heavy in late labour), placental abruption, placenta praevia or rarely, a ruptured uterus or vasa praevia. It should be noted that occasionally placenta praevia remains undiagnosed in pregnancy despite routine and sometimes frequent ultrasound examination.[12]

Resuscitation if required, and diagnosis and management of the cause of bleeding must be the first priorities in dealing with IPH. It is believed to be good practice for protocols to be in place which give clear instructions about how to deal with major obstetric haemorrhage.[6] Practice drills

---

Box 10.3: Risk reduction by the midwife

- Encourage an iron rich diet in pregnancy and consider checking haemoglobin levels through later pregnancy so anaemia is avoided as birth approaches.

- Discuss risk and management issues of the third stage of labour in pregnancy and document the woman's wishes (including whether or not she would consent to a blood transfusion, especially if she is a Jehovah's witness).[12]

- Know the history of each woman supported in labour.

- Know where all equipment is, especially for emergency procedures.

- Thoroughly understand the pathophysiology of the different causes of bleeding, the signs and symptoms, and the most effective treatments.

- Keep labour as normal as possible by offering good psychological support, non-pharmacological pain relief, information, explanations and a listening ear, and encourage the woman to be as upright and active as she is able.

- Where a woman is likely to benefit from intervention, discuss the benefits and risks with her and her partner and listen to her ideas and concerns, to enhance her feeling of emotional well-being and control.

- Make sure she is as involved in decision-making as she is able to be.

- Be aware of the dangers inherent in using prostaglandin, Syntocinon®, unnecessary caesarean section and mismanaging the third stage of labour.

- Be on good terms with your multiprofessional team. Encourage and if necessary lead partnership in decision-making. Be prepared to state a case and be an advocate for the woman.

should be regularly organised for all members of staff based in hospital and the community, and orientation of new staff should include information about how obstetric emergencies are dealt with.

Undiagnosed bleeding in labour

On no account should vaginal examinations or the administration of suppositories or enemas be performed until placenta praevia has been categorically ruled out. These procedures can precipitate torrential haemorrhage.

Initial assessment and management of intrapartum haemorrhage

A woman who starts to bleed heavily *per vaginum* in labour will be extremely concerned both for her own safety and that of her baby. As the midwife deals with the situation, either at home or in hospital, her manner and communication skills will be crucial in enlisting the woman's trust and ultimately her co-operation. The feelings of her partner, if present, must also be taken into consideration.

If the woman's medical and pregnancy histories are not available, the midwife should ascertain these as quickly as possible. If she was not present when the bleeding started, she must also find out the circumstances surrounding the blood loss.

As she collects this information the midwife must also carry out observations on the woman. These include general condition (including pallor, level of consciousness and pain), amount of blood loss, pulse, blood pressure, the nature of any contractions and the condition of the foetus. The midwife will be aware that IPH is unpredictable in its course and the woman's condition may deteriorate rapidly with little or no warning. The midwife must therefore decide in talking to the woman how urgent the need is for a medical or paramedic presence.

Having excluded a normal heavy show in advanced labour and bleeding from haemorrhoids, the midwife must decide whether the woman is having a mild, moderate or severe haemorrhage and on the likely cause. The physiology and management of placental abruption, placenta

praevia and ruptured uterus are discussed in Chapters 5 and 7.

Rarely, vasa praevia may cause IPH. Unlike the previous conditions the mother will not lose blood and so all the signs of this condition will be noted with keen observation and foetal heart rate surveillance. Bleeding will start when the membranes rupture spontaneously or more commonly shortly after their artificial rupture. The mother will not show signs of shock but, unless a speedy diagnosis is made, and the foetus delivered within minutes, it will die through exsanguination. Although intact vasa praevia can be diagnosed by ultrasound in pregnancy, this is not always the case so midwives need to be aware of the condition and that it is more likely to be possible where the placenta is low-lying.

In all cases of IPH if the woman is at home, it is prudent to agree and arrange immediate transfer to hospital, preferably a maternity unit with an on-site, 24-hour haematology unit and blood bank.

The midwife should site an intravenous infusion to open a vein and replace lost fluids. Fluid balance recordings should be commenced.

Having summoned urgent medical aid, management of the labour must continue with basic life support if required, resuscitation, appropriate pain relief and a plan for care.

Management of haemorrhage after the birth and before delivery of the placenta

Intrapartum haemorrhage after the birth of the baby, but before delivery of the placenta is often a midwifery emergency and needs to be dealt with immediately, even if medical aid has been sent for. Bleeding may be from the placental site (uterine atony) where the placenta has wholly or partially separated, or from a cervical or vaginal laceration.

The most common predisposing factors for a partially separated placenta include inco-ordinate action caused by 'fundus fiddling', prolonged labour and precipitate labour.[8] Complicating the condition may be a partial placenta accreta or percreta, where there is morbid adherence of a defective *decidua basalis* with the chorionic villi

---

Box 10.4: Preparation for immediate delivery by caesarean section

- Explain to the woman and her partner what is happening and why.

- Maintain frequent observations, record them and share them.

- Maintain resuscitation procedures until surgery.

- Inform and involve appropriate personnel, including obstetricians, midwives, theatre staff, paediatricians and haematologists.

- Group and cross match blood.

- Routine preparation for surgery, including consent, removal of jewellery and make-up, catheterisation and appropriate local skin care.

---

growing directly into the myometrium or beyond into the perimetrium. However these conditions are rare. Lacerations may complicate any birth, but are more common following instrumental delivery as discussed above or following the birth of a large baby.

Bleeding from a laceration is often obvious. If a vessel can be seen spurting or oozing blood it should be immediately clamped and sutured as soon as possible. Occasionally it is difficult to tell if bleeding is from the uterus, a laceration or both. If the bleeding vessel cannot be located and ligated, and heavy bleeding from the placental bed is suspected, it is prudent to get the placenta delivered as quickly as possible.

Partial separation should be suspected if there is vaginal bleeding with no apparent lengthening of the umbilical cord. Diagnosis is by vaginal examination. If the placenta can be felt just inside the uterine cavity it has separated and should be delivered by controlled cord traction so the cause of the bleeding can be quickly diagnosed and brought under control. However if the fingers can easily be moved into and up the uterus, partial separation is the most likely cause of bleeding.

If the woman has not recently passed urine, the bladder should be emptied. If she does not have an intravenous infusion with Syntocinon® in place, a bolus of 10 units of intravenous Syntocinon® should be administered and nipple stimulation considered, either by putting the baby to the breast or perhaps by the mother rolling her nipples herself. This will encourage natural oxytocin release within seconds and help the mother to feel she is involved in her own recovery.[7]

Enkin and colleagues[16] report that Syntometrine® is more effective in reducing the risk of PPH than oxytocin alone, although it has more unpleasant side effects. However Syntocinon® will contract longitudinal fibres only, not the circular ones around the os, and for this reason, if the woman has started to bleed heavily, Syntometrine® or ergometrine which close the os should be avoided before the placenta has delivered.

The logical conclusion of this information is that Syntometrine® is the drug of choice in active management of the third stage of labour where the woman has given informed consent. However, Syntocinon® is a better drug in managing PPH where the placenta has yet to be expelled through the cervical os. See Box 10.5 for a summary of pharmacological management. Of course the reality in modern British obstetrics is that most women will receive Syntometrine® with the birth of the foetal anterior shoulder and the third stage of their labour will then be actively managed to try to ensure that the placenta is delivered within the five to seven minutes before the ergometrine component of the Syntometrine® closes the os. If the placenta remains partially attached and cannot be removed before the os closes, the birth attendants will need to proceed quickly to a manual removal of the placenta, discussed below, to prevent the blood loss becoming excessive.

Having carried out initial emergency procedures, the midwife should reassess ongoing bleeding and separation of the placenta. If an emergency situation persists and the baby has been born at home, transfer to hospital must be arranged. However it is always preferable to

Box 10.5: Pharmacological methods of managing atony

Intramuscular, intravenous bolus or intravenous infusion (IVI) of Syntocinon®

Given intramuscularly Syntocinon® takes 2½ minutes to act on the uterus and given intravenously, within 45 seconds. In acute primary PPH, 5 units should be given by slow intravenous injection, followed up by 5–20 more units added to 500 ml intravenous solution and run into the vein at a rate sufficient to control uterine atony. This is the manufacturer's recommended dose but in practice women may be given up to 40 units in 500 ml of intravenous fluid. Fluid overload must be avoided as this has inherent dangers. High doses of Syntocinon® can cause nausea, vomiting, arrhythmias, rash and anaphylactic reactions including hypotension.

Intramuscular Syntometrine® (5 units oxytocin and 0.5 mg ergometrine)

Syntometrine® is a drug of choice in British obstetrics as it can be prescribed by the midwife and has a more sustained action than Syntocinon® alone. It will act on the uterus within 2½ minutes causing a prolonged contraction. No more than two doses should be administered because the ergometrine component can cause severe peripheral vasoconstriction, a sharp rise in blood pressure and pulmonary hypertension. For these reasons it should never be administered to women with high blood pressure or severe asthma. It is also contra-indicated in women with heart, liver and renal disease and some other medical disorders. Side effects include nausea and vomiting.

Intramuscular, intravenous bolus or intrauterine injection of ergometrine (0.25–0.5 mg)

Ergometrine can be given intramuscularly, intravenously or directly into uterine muscle. Given intramuscularly, ergometrine takes 2½ minutes to act and given intravenously, up to 45 seconds. If it is injected into uterine muscle it will take effect almost immediately although this route of administration is rarely seen in practice. The midwife must not administer more than two doses of 0.5 mg ergometrine intramuscularly or intravenously, and the same contra-indications as for Syntometrine® apply.

Intramuscular carboprost tromethamine (Hemabate®) (250 µg in 1 ml)

Carboprost is a type of prostaglandin which causes contraction of the myometrium to treat atony. It is often given when Syntometrine® and/or Syntocinon® have been ineffective and up to 8 doses can be given, no closer than 15 minutes apart and more usually with an hour and a half between doses. It can potentiate the effect of oxytocin and when both have been used, the woman should be closely monitored. Carboprost should never be given intravenously or to women with hypertension, severe asthma, pelvic inflammatory disease, cardiac, pulmonary, renal or hepatic disease. This drug is not normally accessible at a home birth.

deliver the placenta before transferring a woman by ambulance and every effort should be made to do so. It is highly dangerous to move a woman who is bleeding heavily from a partially separated placenta.

If it has not already been done, the midwife should now consider siting an intravenous infusion. This must be done before accessible veins in the arms collapse, which would make the procedure more difficult and more time-consuming. Community-based midwives should be proficient in intravenous cannulation and hospital-based midwives will also find it advantageous to have this skill, especially as more birth centres are likely to be set up in the UK in the near future.[17] An intravenous opening can then be used to replace lost fluid and may be useful for adding drugs as necessary.

If bleeding continues, manual removal of the placenta should now be considered (*see* Box 10.6 and Figure 10.1). Although a very simple procedure, it is a painful one for the mother and

---

Box 10.6: Manual removal of the placenta

- Observe strict aseptic technique.

- Use elbow-length gloves.

- Insert a whole hand through the os following the cord (if it is still attached to the placenta), while the other hand supports the fundus to prevent it being pushed upwards.

- Slip the internal hand between the separated portion of the placenta and the wall of the uterus and gently prise the placenta off with a spatula-like movement, moving the hand smoothly back and forth.

- Once it has been separated, manually sweep all fragments of placenta from the placental site.

- Grasp the placenta and manually remove it from the uterus.

- Once the removal has been completed, the uterus should be vigorously massaged to rub up a contraction.

---

carries a risk of infection and uterine rupture if performed too roughly. Accordingly the procedure is only suitable in an emergency, although the *Midwives Rules and Code of Practice*[18] state that the midwife must be able to perform this manoeuvre in such an emergency. The course of action must be explained to the parents and the partner given the opportunity to leave the room, perhaps to care for the baby, if desired.

Syntocinon® should be given, preferably by continuous intravenous infusion, as soon as the placenta is out and this will be continued for a few hours. If the woman is still at home, it may be more appropriate to give ergometrine to aid contraction of the uterus before transfer to hospital. The placenta is quickly examined for completeness, and if there is any doubt an evacuation of the uterus (ERPC) should be considered in hospital. Blood loss must be measured and recorded, and contemporaneous notes made. If she is still at home, the woman should be transferred to hospital whether or not she shows signs of shock, in case of uterine muscle relaxation in the next 24 hours. The placenta should also be sent to hospital with the woman, so the obstetricians can make their own decision about its completeness and suggest future management for the woman. She will almost certainly be offered a full blood count to check for anaemia and antibiotics because of her increased risk of uterine infection. Close observation of both the mother and the baby should be continued during this time.

Occasionally a partially separated placenta cannot be completely removed manually because it is morbidly adherent to the uterine wall. If the midwife suspects this is the case at a home birth, she should administer an oxytocic if there is any blood loss, with the aim of minimising it while transfer to hospital is made.

Management of haemorrhage after delivery of the placenta

Elizabeth Davis[8] comments that the slow, steady trickle of blood after delivery of the placenta can be the most dangerous of all if it is not closely monitored. Changes of shift, failure to add up the total blood loss and frequent changes of the bed sheets may lead midwives to underestimate the situation and the woman may slowly sink into unconsciousness while the midwife completes her record-keeping.

The causes of excessive bleeding after delivery of the placenta tend to be the same as for bleeding before its delivery, namely lacerations or atonic uterus. If there is a continuous gush of blood, the midwife must immediately diagnose the cause of the heavy bleeding. There may or may not have been excessive bleeding before the delivery of the placenta and the present cause of bleeding may or may not remain the same. Continual assessment of the situation is therefore necessary.

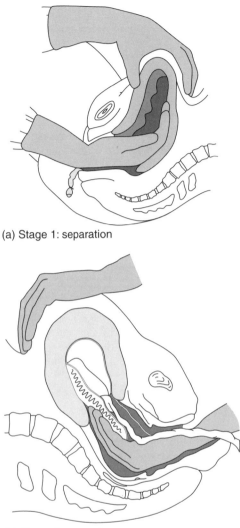

(a) Stage 1: separation

(b) Stage 2: removal

Figure 10.1 Manual removal of placenta

Lacerations incurred during the birth of the baby may only now become apparent as a significant cause of bleeding, as expeditious delivery of the placenta may have preoccupied the midwife until now. If the uterus is well contracted, haemostasis needs to be quickly achieved and lacerations sutured. If the woman is at home, the midwife must consider how best to position her and how to achieve optimal lighting, especially if she has not had the opportunity to do this during the woman's pregnancy (for instance in a case of unplanned home birth). This may require some ingenuity on the midwife's part. However it is vital that she isolates the apex of the laceration, repairing it speedily and adequately before the blood loss compromises the well-being of the woman.

If atonic uterus is diagnosed in this situation its cause may remain unknown. However of the known causes, retention of placental tissue, membrane or blood clot interfering with contraction of the myometrium are the most likely. Retained products can sometimes be diagnosed from examination of the expelled placenta and membranes, but this is by no means foolproof. Clots in the uterus should be suspected if the placenta and membranes appear to be complete, the uterus feels enlarged and a little soft, and a slow trickle of blood after placental delivery gradually increases. A full bladder should also be considered if the bladder has not been emptied recently or the woman has had a high fluid intake (oral or intravenous).

Many predisposing factors to PPH, such as multiple birth, polyhydramnios, antepartum haemorrhage or instrumental delivery will have already led to the attendance of an obstetrician. However if uterine atony is diagnosed and a doctor is not present, the midwife should immediately summon medical aid, explain what is happening to the woman and her birth partner, tell them briefly what she is going to do and ask for their co-operation. The woman needs to get into a semi-recumbent or recumbent position preferably on a bed. The uterus should be made to contract as soon as possible by the following means.

- Rub up a contraction (*see* Box 10.7 and Figure 10.2). This may also express offending blood clots.

- Catheterise the bladder. Any urine deposited may interfere with strong contraction and at this point the midwife needs to know that the bladder is empty and kept empty until the bleeding is brought under control.

- Consider a (further) dose of Syntocinon® as an intravenous bolus or by infusion, or Syntometrine® intramuscularly (if the woman is normotensive).

- If the woman is able to put the baby to the breast this will release natural oxytocin which will promote uterine muscle contraction.

Box 10.7: Rubbing up a contraction

- Gently feel for the fundus with the pads of the fingertips (a manoeuvre similar to palpation of the fundus in pregnancy) and assess uterine contraction. A right-handed midwife standing on the woman's right side will do this with the left hand.

- Cup the hand around the uterus and massage it firmly but gently (this action should not be painful for the woman) with a smooth, circular movement until its soft texture starts to become firmer with an oncoming contraction.

- Hold the hand still and do not recommence massage unless the uterus starts to relax again.

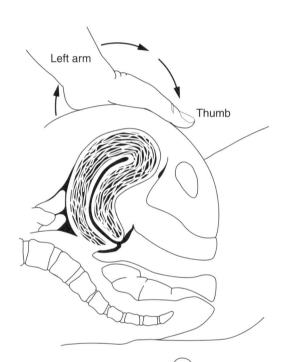

The left hand is cupped over the uterus ( ) and massages it with a firm circular motion in a clockwise direction.

Figure 10.2 Rubbing up a contraction

These measures will bring many cases of haemorrhage from atony speedily under control. However, if bleeding is becoming potentially life-threatening, the midwife should perform bi-manual compression (*see* Figure 10.3).

To achieve bi-manual compression one hand is placed in the anterior fornix of the vagina and clenched, while the other hand massages the fundus, thereby pressing the walls of the uterus together. Alternatively, bi-manual compression can be done externally by grasping the uterus with both hands and squashing the uterus between them.[8] It should be noted that internal bi-manual compression in particular is extremely painful for the woman and should only be performed if other procedures are not effective, while await-ing medical action. Needless to say all this should be explained clearly to the woman and her partner before the procedure is attempted, as great distress will be caused if either is

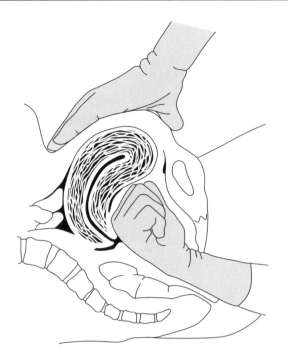

Figure 10.3 Internal bi-manual compression

unprepared for the extreme discomfort which will ensue.

If these procedures do not work, the midwife and any other health professionals who have been summoned, should consider a blood coagulation problem. Urgent blood tests will be done to enable diagnosis and the correct management. The mother is now likely to be shocked and should be treated with intravenous fluids and appropriate drugs. A central venous line may be indicated and a blood transfusion ordered. Bi-manual compression will need to be continued until the bleeding is brought under control.

A blood coagulation problem is relatively easy to diagnose because bleeding continues either in a steady stream or a gush and does not clot where it collects. Once medical diagnosis has been made and haematological results are known to ascertain the extent of the problem, it can be treated accordingly.

In all cases of continued bleeding, uterine packing may be considered. Dry sterile gauze is used, which can be moistened with saline.[19] Analgesia is required during the procedure and antibiotic cover is suggested. A bladder catheter should remain *in situ* for 24–36 hours until the

pack is removed on the delivery suite, with operating facilities at the ready in case bleeding restarts. Park and Sachs[19] however suggest that laparotomy to discover the direct cause of bleeding may be more suitable.

Less common treatments, which have been attempted with varying success in the control of PPH and in which the midwife may be called upon to assist the medical practitioner, include insertion of a Sengstaken-Blakemore tube or Foyeys catheter into the uterus, inflation of the balloon and external compression of the uterus for ten minutes; ligation of the internal iliac artery; direct ligation of the uterine vessels; uterine devascularisation and the use of uterine compression sutures. These are described by Drife[20] in a review of management techniques for primary PPH.

A uterine artery embolisation may be attempted[21] and although this appears to be an effective way of avoiding hysterectomy in intractable haemorrhage, the necessity of performing the procedure under radiological guidance makes it impractical in many maternity units.

As a final attempt to stop the bleeding in the unlikely event of all else failing, the woman will

---

Box 10.8: Diagnosis and management of disseminated intravascular coagulopathy

Diagnosis

- An acute history of a predisposing condition (e.g. placental abruption).

- Bleeding from orifices, e.g. nose, mouth, venepuncture site, haematuria.

- Blood loss does not immediately clot.

- Torrential haemorrhage.

- Signs of circulatory obstruction, e.g. cyanosis in fingers, cerebrovascular accident (stroke) or renal failure.

- Blood test results: low haemoglobin, abnormal clotting study results (prothrombin time, abnormal levels of platelets, fibrinogen and FDPs).

- Prompt diagnosis and management are vital for maternal survival.

Management

- Refer to the local protocol, which should be drawn up on how DIC should be managed.

- Request urgent medical attendance when DIC is suspected.

- Look for the underlying cause if it is not known (DIC is never a primary disease) although the woman's condition will be stabilised before the condition is treated (or the baby delivered, when the condition occurs in pregnancy).

- Give explanations and emotional support to the woman and her partner as necessary.

- Urgent blood test results will dictate the course of management, including full blood count, clotting studies and time taken to group and cross match blood. Replacement of blood cells and clotting factors will be required with fresh frozen plasma, platelet concentrates and ultimately, with red blood cells.

- Maintain frequent and accurate observations of the woman's vital signs. The bladder should be catheterised and fluid balance vigilantly monitored. Any sign of renal failure must be reported to the team immediately.

---

be taken to the operating theatre for close investigation of her uterus and its blood vessels. In severe cases of uncontrollable bleeding, hysterectomy will be performed to save the woman's life.

Conclusion

Peripartum haemorrhage in the mother is the obstetric emergency the midwife is most likely to face in her career. Many potential cases can be and are avoided by skilled support of women throughout pregnancy and in labour. A significant number of actual cases can be predicted from women's histories and with the appropriate use of technology. Wherever possible, management options should be discussed with the woman to ensure that she is involved in decision-making about her care. A minority of cases of obstetric haemorrhage occur without warning and the midwife, along with the multiprofessional obstetric team, need to be equipped to deal with these situations, whether at home or in hospital.

With prompt and skilful management, the majority of intrapartum and early postpartum haemorrhages can be brought under control with a minimum of interventions.

References

1 American Academy of Family Physicians (1996) *Advanced Life Support in Obstetrics.* American Academy of Family Physicians, Newcastle Upon Tyne.

2 Cruikshank DP, Wigton TR and Hayes PM (1996) Maternal physiology in pregnancy. In: SG Gabbe, JR Niebyl and JL Simpson (eds) *Obstetrics: normal and problem pregnancies* (3e). Churchill Livingstone, New York.

3 Levy V and Moore J (1985) The midwife's management of the third stage of labour. *Nurs Times.* **81** (5): 47–50.

4 Prendiville WJ, Elbourne DR and Chalmers I (1988) The Bristol third stage trial: active versus physiological management of the third stage of labour. *BMJ.* **297**: 1295–300.

5 Waterstone M, Bewley S and Wolfe C (2001) Incidence and predictors of severe obstetric morbidity: case control study. *BMJ.* **322**: 1089–94.

6 Lewis G (ed) (2001) *Why Mothers Die 1997–1999: the fifth report of the confidential enquiries into maternal deaths in the United Kingdom.* RCOG Press, London.

7 Stables D (1999) *Physiology of Childbearing.* Baillière Tindall, London.

8 Davis E (1997) *Hearts and Hands.* Celestial Arts, Berkeley.

9 Benedetti TJ (1996) Obstetric hemorrhage. In: SG Gabbe, JR Niebyl and JL Simpson (eds) *Obstetrics: normal and problem pregnancies* (3e). Churchill Livingstone, New York.

10 Coulter-Smith SD, Holohan M and Darling MRN (1996) Previous caesarean section: a risk factor for major obstetric haemorrhage? *J Obstet Gynaecol.* **16** (5): 349–52.

11 Goer H (1995) Obstetric Myths Versus Research Realities. Bergin and Garvey, Westport.

12 Department of Health (1998) *Why Mothers Die: report on confidential enquiries into maternal deaths in the United Kingdom 1994–1996.* The Stationery Office, London.

13 Bofill JA, Rust OA, Devidas M et al. (1996) Prognostic factors for moderate and severe maternal genital tract laceration with operative vaginal delivery. *Am J Obstet Gynecol.* **174**: 353.

14 Evans W and Edelstone DI (2000) Instrumental delivery. In: LH Kean, PN Baker and DI Edelstone (eds) *Best Practice in Labor Ward Management.* WB Saunders, Edinburgh.

15 McDonald S (1999) Physiology and management of the third stage of labour. In: VR Bennett and LK Brown (eds) *Myles Textbook for Midwives.* Churchill Livingstone, Edinburgh.

16 Enkin M, Keirse MJNC, Neilson J et al. (2000) *A Guide to Effective Care in Pregnancy and Labour.* Oxford University Press, Oxford.

17 Rosser J (2001) Birth centres across the UK: a win/win strategy for saving normal birth. *RCM Midwives J.* **4** (3): 88–9.

18 United Kingdom Central Council for Nursing, Midwifery and Health Visiting (1998) Midwives Rules and Code of Practice. UKCC, London.

19 Park EH and Sachs BP (1999) Postpartum haemorrhage and other problems of the third stage. In: DK James, PJ Steer, CP Weiner and B Gonik (eds) *High Risk Pregnancy: management options.* WB Saunders, London.

20 Drife J (1997) Management of primary postpartum haemorrhage. *Br J Obstet Gynaecol.* **104** (3): 275–7.

21 Vedantham S, Goodwin SC, McLucas B et al. (1997) Uterine artery embolization: an underused method of controlling pelvic hemorrhage. *Am J Obstet Gynecol.* **176** (4): 938–48.

CHAPTER 11

Other causes of potential maternal collapse

Maureen Boyle

This chapter considers the less common causes of maternal conditions which need emergency or urgent attention. It should be noted that all of these conditions fall outside the midwife's remit and therefore her role is to provide a high standard of supportive care after summoning emergency assistance or organising urgent referral.

For most of these conditions prompt medical or surgical aid is the only treatment. However it could be that an overview of the potential causes of the woman's symptoms will help the midwife to decide how best to support her, especially in isolated situations, until assistance arrives. It is also possible that prior revision of these conditions will lead to earlier suspicion and referral of symptoms which might otherwise have progressed to an emergency situation. Knowledge of these conditions may also be useful if the midwife wishes to continue her duty of care and act as the woman's advocate.[1]

The overview given here is of necessity very brief and is intended to be just a summary. However, it will provide a starting point before accessing other resources for more in-depth information. Further information may also be necessary in preparation for discussing the situation with a woman who has suffered any of these conditions.

The main presenting symptoms of maternal collapse are identified in the first part of this chapter, with the conditions that may be the potential cause listed alphabetically below each one. Of course many conditions manifest with various symptoms, depending on the degree of severity or just the individual aetiology and therefore may appear in more than one list. Some of these conditions are discussed in previous chapters. Others are briefly summarised later in this chapter, presented in alphabetical order. All require urgent care.

Loss of consciousness

A useful assessment tool when evaluating level of consciousness is the Glasgow Coma Score given in Table 11.1.

Table 11.1: The Glasgow Coma Score

Response	Level of response	Score
Eye opening	Spontaneous	4
	To speech	3
	To pain	2
	Nil	1
Motor response	Obeys command	6
	Localises pain	5
	Normal flexion to pain	4
	Abnormal flexion to pain	3
	Abnormal extension	2
	Nil	1
Verbal response	Orientated	5
	Confused	4
	Inappropriate	3
	Incomprehensible	2
	Nil	1

A woman with a score of less than eight is in a coma and probably needs respiratory support. If the score falls two or more points, this represents a significant deterioration in neurological condition.

A diagnosis of amniotic fluid embolism (*see* Chapter 7) should be considered at an early stage in all cases of unexplained maternal collapse.[2]

Common causes

- Acute (adult) respiratory distress syndrome (ARDS) (*see* page 129).
- Amniotic fluid embolism (*see* Chapter 7).
- Anaphylaxis (*see* page 130).
- Aneurysm: ruptured.
- Asthma (*see* page 131).
- Cerebrovascular accident or stroke (*see* page 131).
- Diabetic ketoacidosis (*see* page 131).
- Drug intoxication.
- Epidural: high block (*see* page 132).
- Eclampsia (*see* Chapter 4).
- Haematoma: paravaginal or paragenital (*see* page 132).
- Hyperventilation.
- Hypoglycaemia (*see* page 132).
- Hypotension.
- Local anaesthetic toxicity.
- Magnesium toxicity (*see* Chapter 4).
- Myocardial infarction.
- Peripartum cardiomyopathy (*see* page 133).
- Pulmonary embolism (*see* Chapter 3).
- Thyroid crisis (*see* page 134).
- Uterine rupture (*see* Chapter 8).

Chest pain

Because heartburn is so common a complaint in pregnancy, chest pain may not be treated with the urgency it may need in some rare cases. However, life-threatening causes usually present with severe pain, unrelieved by common medicine, and are associated with other symptoms (for example, dyspnoea, nausea, vomiting and altered consciousness). A lesson can be learned from a case in the *Report on Confidential Enquiries into Maternal Deaths*[3] concerning a woman of 33 weeks' gestation who, after seeking repeat antacids from her GP and seemingly with no other signs than proteinurea and some oedema, died suddenly at home from eclampsia.

Common causes

- Aortic dissection.
- Myocardial infarction.
- Pericarditis.
- Peripartum cardiomyopathy (*see* page 133).
- Pleurisy.
- Pneumonia.
- Pneumothorax.
- Pre-eclampsia: fulminating (*see* Chapter 4).
- Pulmonary embolism (*see* Chapter 3).
- Sickle-cell crisis (*see* page 134).

Confusion

Confusion may manifest not only as inappropriate speech, but also as withdrawal of communication or aggression. The midwife must make a decision on whether the cause could be a pathophysiological condition before deciding on the most appropriate action.

Common causes

- ARDS (*see* page 129).
- Asthma (*see* page 131).
- Cerebrovascular accident (*see* page 131).
- Drug intoxication or drug withdrawal.
- Hypoglycaemia (*see* page 132).
- Hypotension.
- Hypoxia.

- Magnesium toxicity (*see* Chapter 4).

- Permanent mental disability.

- Pre-eclampsia: fulminating (*see* Chapter 4).

- Psychiatric illness.

- Pulmonary oedema (*see* page 133).

- Sepsis (*see* page 133).

- Thyroid crisis (*see* page 134).

Shock

See Chapter 2 for a full discussion on the signs, symptoms and related pathophysiology of shock.

Common causes

- ARDS (*see* page 129).

- Amniotic fluid embolism (*see* Chapter 7).

- Antepartum haemorrhage (*see* Chapter 5).

- Appendicitis (*see* page 130).

- Ectopic pregnancy (*see* page 131).

- Postpartum haemorrhage (*see* Chapter 10).

- Pulmonary embolism (*see* Chapter 3).

- Sepsis (*see* page 133).

- Uterine inversion (*see* Chapter 8).

- Uterine rupture (*see* Chapter 8).

Abdominal pain

Common causes

- Antepartum haemorrhage (*see* Chapter 5).

- Appendicitis (*see* page 130).

- Ectopic pregnancy (*see* page 131).

- Fibroids (*see* page 132).

- Haematoma: rectus (*see* page 132).

- Pyelonephritis.

- Renal stones (unusual in pregnancy as the renal tract is dilated).

- Thyroid crisis (*see* page 134).

- Uterine inversion (*see* Chapter 8).

- Uterine rupture (*see* Chapter 8).

Convulsion

Common causes

- Eclampsia (*see* Chapter 4).

- Amniotic fluid embolism (*see* Chapter 7).

- Epilepsy.

- Sickle-cell crisis (*see* page 134).

Trauma

It is always possible that a midwife may be the first person on the scene following a car accident, a violent incident or other injury to a pregnant woman. In these circumstances it is possible to do no more than provide skilled first aid, remembering that the best way to care for the foetus is to adequately resuscitate the mother (*see* Chapter 2). After calling for emergency help, initial assessment and action should include the emergency measures in Box 11.1.

Acute (adult) respiratory distress syndrome

ARDS is usually the result of another condition (for example, amniotic fluid embolism, acute infection, eclampsia, abruption or anaphylaxis)[4] and although mortality has been quoted as high as 50%, for the survivors the long-term prognosis is good with lung function recovery back to normal in four to six months in many women.[5] However there are also the possibilities of complications of ventilation and admission to an intensive therapy unit.

Women will show signs of acute respiratory distress such as tachycardia, tachyapnoea and cyanosis. There will be lung crackles and bilateral interstitial infiltrates appear on chest x-ray.[6] Diagnosis is by clinical signs, but the primary cause also needs to be diagnosed and treated concurrently.

Box 11.1: Emergency care

- Airway: maintain open. Ensure a lateral tilt or displace the uterus, while protecting the cervical and remainder of the spine.

- Breathing: assist if necessary.

- Circulation: control obvious bleeding if possible and give cardiac massage if necessary.

- Disability: assess level of consciousness by noting response to voice or pain.

- Environment: keep warm and safe.

Treatment, usually in an intensive care unit, is aimed at treating the cause and supporting lung function until the lung heals.[7] Optimum oxygenation must be maintained and acidosis, anaemia and hypothermia prevented.[8] Careful fluid balance is necessary to prevent pulmonary oedema and ventilation may be necessary.

Anaphylaxis

Anaphylaxis is an acute response, with multi-system involvement resulting from the rapid release of inflammatory mediators, to a substance to which the woman has become sensitised. The substance may commonly be a drug, food or a material such as latex. The response usually begins rapidly within seconds or minutes and a full reaction occurs within 30 minutes.

Possible signs and symptoms include urticaria, pruritus, flushing, erythema, nausea, vomiting and diarrhoea, tachycardia, laryngeal oedema, generalised oedema, bronchospasm, hypotension and respiratory or cardiac collapse.

The treatment is to stop any drugs and infusions etc., administer oxygen and monitor oxygen saturations, obtain intravenous (IV) access and administer fluids to maintain blood pressure. Blood gases must be monitored and full blood counts and clotting studies carried out. An electrocardiograph (ECG) and x-ray may be necessary. Depending on the woman's condition, a left lateral tilt may be the optimum position, and intubation and ventilation for respiratory support may be necessary.

Drug therapy is an important part of treatment and may include epinephrine, antihistamines, corticosteroids and bronchodilators.

If the woman is still pregnant, cardiotocography (CTG) monitoring is appropriate and delivery may be needed, although foetal distress may be a response to maternal hypoxia and hypotension, and resolve as she is treated.

If a woman has had a suspected anaphylactic reaction, it needs investigating usually by a local allergy clinic.

Latex allergy is apparently increasing, so midwives need to suspect this cause and possibly anticipate it by asking specific questions (perhaps at booking) regarding women's previous reactions to other latex products such as condoms, balloons or household rubber gloves.[9] If latex allergy is identified, great care is needed because much of normal midwifery equipment (such as tape, catheters, masks, etc. as well as gloves) contain latex.

Appendicitis

Appendicitis is relatively common in pregnant women, occuring in approximately one in 1600 pregnant women. It may be harder to diagnose in pregnancy because the gravid uterus displaces the appendix, so the pain may be higher and more lateral although right lower quadrant pain is still the most common presenting symptom at any gestational age.[10,11] In addition, because of the change of position of the appendix, peritonitis is a more common complication in pregnant women.[12]

Signs and symptoms may include pain, nausea, vomiting and maybe pyrexia.

Treatment is surgical and necessary at any stage of pregnancy. A delay in diagnosis and treatment can lead to perforation and/or peritonitis and potentially to maternal and foetal morbidity or mortality.[13]

Asthma

Asthma affects 0.4–1.3% of pregnancies and is the most common obstructive pulmonary disorder occurring during pregnancy.[14,15] The effect of pregnancy on asthma is unpredictable, but a history of asthma does seem to predispose the woman to an increased likelihood of other complications of pregnancy.[16]

Signs and symptoms of an asthma attack may include increased respiration rate, increased heart rate, use of accessory muscles for breathing and bronchospasm. As the attack worsens in severity, the woman may make only a poor respiratory effort, become exhausted, cyanosed, confused and finally bradycardic and comatosed.

Treatment includes the administration of humidified oxygen, intravenous access and fluids, drug therapy with bronchodilators or systemic steroids and on-going assessment with pulse oximeter, ECG, x-ray, arterial blood gases, maternal peak flow and CTG if antenatal. With a severe asthma attack that is difficult to treat (status asthmaticus) and progressing to respiratory failure, intubation and ventilation are needed.[17]

Cerebrovascular accident

Although considered a condition of old age, strokes happen to childbearing women: one American study of 89 913 deliveries reported an incidence of 1:6000 pregnancies.[18] It seems that although the risk of stroke is not increased during pregnancy, women are at increased risk in the six weeks following delivery.[19]

Just under 50% of cerebrovascular accidents (CVAs) in childbearing women are associated with eclampsia.[20] A stroke may be either ischaemic or haemorrhagic and symptoms are similar although treatments will differ. An ischaemic stroke is caused by severe loss of blood flow to part of the brain; in young women, a cardioembolism is a common cause. This may be limited and cause only a transient ischaemic attack (TIA) or it may be prolonged and cause permanent damage or death. Most TIAs and about 25% of ischaemic strokes happen in the first postpartum week.[21] A haemorrhagic stroke is caused by a bleed, either intracerebral or subarachnoid, and may result from a vessel wall or other haematological abnormality.

Symptoms can range in severity from headache and mild muscle weakness to collapse and cardio or respiratory arrest.

Various investigations may be needed to determine a diagnosis, including computed tomography (CT scan), magnetic resonance imaging (MRI), lumbar puncture and haematological testing.

Treatment of ischaemic stroke includes possible anticoagulation, while treatment of haemorrhagic stroke is usually surgical. On-going treatment needs will depend on the severity of the stroke.

Diabetic ketoacidosis

Diabetic ketoacidosis is a medical emergency affecting about 1–3% of diabetic pregnancies and has the potential for maternal mortality. However, improvement in the care of pregnant diabetic women has reduced this risk. Nevertheless, foetal mortality remains high.[22]

Diabetic ketoacidosis normally affects only those with type I diabetes, but it is not unknown in type II. In fact, a recent *Report on Confidential Enquiries into Maternal Deaths*[3] included the postnatal death of a woman considered to have had gestational diabetes, so attention to follow-up care is clearly necessary. The most common cause of diabetic ketoacidosis is infection, although pyrexia may not be present.[22]

Diabetic ketoacidosis can present as a collapse (coma) but may be preceded by excessive thirst, polyuria, abdominal pain, vomiting, hyperventilation and/or weakness.

Diagnosis is usually by arterial pH: a dipstick of urine may show 4+ glucose. However, in pregnancy a woman may have significant ketoacidosis with only slight serum hyperglycaemia.[23]

Treatment includes appropriate resuscitation, then rehydration, careful blood glucose monitoring and glucose or insulin therapy as necessary. Infection must be investigated and treated.

Reduced variability and decelerations on the CTG will often resolve, with improvement of the maternal condition, so caesarean section for foetal distress is not usually necessary.[24]

Ectopic pregnancy

Ectopic pregnancies are a common complication. The majority of them occur as a singleton pregnancy within the fallopian tubes. However the occurrence of heterotopic pregnancy, a combination of ectopic and intrauterine pregnancy, is increasing and is probably due to the increase in assisted conceptions.[25]

Abdominal pain is usually felt from about four to six weeks. However pain may be referred and it has been stated that pain anywhere from shoulder to knee in sexually active women of childbearing age should be assessed for ectopic pregancy.[26] Rupture and vaginal bleeding may occur from five to ten weeks, and be accompanied by nausea and vomiting.

Diagnosis is by positive pregnancy test and abdominal or vaginal ultrasound.

Treatment involves resuscitation as necessary to stabilise the woman's condition, including administering IV fluids, including blood, and laparascopic or abdominal surgery. In an early and unruptured ectopic pregnancy, it may be possible to treat the condition medically.[27]

Epidural: high block

In an Australian study of 10 995 epidurals, high blocks occured on eight occasions (0.07%) and two of these women required intubation and ventilation.[28]

High blocks may occur as a result of an unexpected spread of local anaesthetic after a subarachnoid (spinal) injection or after an accidental subarachnoid injection of an epidural dose of local anaesthetic.

Signs and symptoms are dependent on the height of the block but may include tingling, weakness in hands, different breathing, hypotension and/or bradycardia. With a total spinal block, loss of consciousness will occur due to the direct action of local anaesthetic on the brain.

Immediate treatment is to turn off the epidural if running as a continuous infusion and commence resuscitation if necessary. Anaesthetists will treat hypotension and bradycardia as appropriate. The CTG will reflect the mother's condition but adequate resuscitation and treatment should maintain foetal well-being.

Fibroids

Fibroids are common benign tumours which can be located in the uterus. In pregnancy, they may degrade (usually causing dark red or brown vaginal loss), stay the same or grow in which case

they may compromise the growth of the foetus or cause premature labour. If they are positioned low down in the uterus, they may interfere with the lie and descent into the pelvis of the foetus, and subsequently with the mode of birth.

These conditions are not usually acute in the antenatal period, although fibroids may be a cause of postpartum haemorrhage (*see* Chapter 10). However if peduncular, a fibroid may twist (torsion) which could cause acute abdominal pain, vomiting and pyrexia. Diagnosis is usually by ultrasound, and surgery may be necessary.

Haematoma: paravaginal or paragenital

If a woman collapses or shows signs of shock after the third stage and there is no visible sign of haemorrhage, a concealed haemorrhage may be suspected.[29]

Although it would be expected that most severe genital tract trauma would be caused by an instrumental delivery, the most recent *Report on Confidential Enquiries into Maternal Deaths*[30] includes the case of a woman giving birth to a preterm baby unattended and subsequently dying from a vaginal wall haematoma, despite treatment.

Treatment is resuscitation as necessary, including siting an IV, and treating the cause. Depending on the site, the haematoma may be treated through the vagina or the woman may need a laparotomy.

Haematoma: rectus

This is a rare condition and occurs when a sudden spasm such as a sneeze ruptures the inferior epigastric veins and/or causes the rectus muscle to dehisce. This usually only takes place late in pregnancy when the abdominal wall is under pressure from a large uterus.[10]

Signs and symptoms include severe local pain and possible slight blood loss. Diagnosis is usually from symptoms, but ultrasound may be used.

Treatment will depend on the severity and may be conservative or surgical.

Hypoglycaemia

Hypoglycaemia can cause rapid loss of consciousness in contrast to diabetic ketoacidosis which causes gradual loss of consciousness. It can be immediately life-threatening.

Hypoglycaemia can present not only in diabetes mellitus, but also in Addison's disease, hypopituitarism and hypothyroidism. Diagnosis is by measurement of the blood glucose.

Treatment includes resuscitation as necessary and, following assessment of blood glucose, IV administration of 50% dextrose or glucagon given intramuscularly if no IV access is possible. This should be accompanied by oxygen administration, oxygen saturation monitoring, and, if antenatal, CTG monitoring of the foetal well-being.

Peripartum cardiomyopathy

Peripartum cardiomyopathy is suspected when congestive cardiac failure develops in a previously fit woman towards the end of pregnancy or within about five months postnatally. Aetiology is unknown but may be a myocarditis caused by infection or an autoimmune response.[31] The rate of maternal mortality can be about 25–50%.

Risk factors include advanced maternal age, multiparity, twin pregnancy, long-term tocolytic therapy and perhaps cocaine abuse.

Presenting signs and symptoms may include dyspnoea, tachyapnoea, cough, orthopnoea, palpitations, tachycardia, haemoptysis, chest pain, abdominal pain, ascites, periferal oedema and/or confusion.

A cardiac assessment is needed and peripartum cardiomyopathy is diagnosed after exclusion of other causes of cardiac failure. Treatment involves care by a cardiology team in a cardiac unit, with close monitoring and support of cardiac and respiratory function. If the woman is still pregnant, delivery should be expedited.

Early diagnosis is vital to ensure optimum outcome, but there may never be a full recovery.[31,32] If the condition persists for more than six months, it is associated with a poor outcome.

There is uncertainty as to whether peripartum cardiomyopathy will reoccur in a future pregnancy, but studies have demonstrated a poor outcome.[33]

Pulmonary oedema

Pulmonary oedema is a potential complication of many conditions including pre-eclampsia, septicaemia, pulmonary embolism, amniotic fluid embolism or it may be caused by fluid overload and/or tocolytic treatment for premature labour.[5]

Fluid may enter the alveoli of the lungs due to pulmonary capillary damage or may diffuse from the vessels due to a reduction in colloid oncotic pressure.[34] This fluid will not only block effective oxygenation, but also damage the alveoli.

The woman will appear breathless, tachycardic and may have haemoptysis. Diagnosis will be made on clinical signs and x-ray findings, and treatment includes respiratory support as necessary, drugs including diuretics in particular, and careful fluid balance monitoring. Pulmonary oedema must be effectively treated or it may progress to ARDS.

Sepsis

Although infection during or after pregnancy is a relatively common condition, it is not normally serious because childbearing women are usually young and healthy, and in the UK, infections are identified and treated. However, eighteen women died of sepsis before or after delivery in a recent *Report into Confidential Enquiries into Maternal Deaths*.[30] These cases demonstrate that early signs may not always be easily recognised and that a fulminating septicaemia can occur rapidly.

An infected woman may be pyrexial, but this may progress to hypothermia in septic shock. Her skin may change from warm and dry, to red and clammy. She will be tachycardic and confusion may be present relatively early in the process. Severe sepsis can cause organ dysfunction, hypotension despite adequate fluid intake or administration, and hypoperfusion.

Diagnosis of the source of infection is necessary. Relevant specimens (for example, urine and wound drainage) must be collected and cultured. Blood cultures should be obtained when a woman is most pyrexial, but note that less than half of patients with septic shock have positive blood cultures.[35] A chest x-ray, ultrasound or CT scan may be appropriate and the woman may need surgery for diagnosis.

Treatment will depend on the symptoms and the woman's condition, but will involve appropriate respiratory support, antibiotics and careful monitoring of vital signs, general condition and fluid balance. She may also need surgery for drainage and/or debridement.

In the worst cases sepsis could lead to acute renal failure, respiratory failure and/or DIC.

Sickle-cell crisis

A sickle-cell crisis is more common in pregnancy because of increased hypercoagulability, especially in the third trimester and following birth. About one third of pregnant women with sickle-cell disease will have at least one pain crisis.[36] Care must be taken to ensure that the pain is not from a cause unrelated to the disease, for example abruption, pulmonary embolism, or fulminating pre-eclampsia. The pregnant woman with sickle-cell disease is at high risk for pre-eclampsia.[37]

Signs and symptoms will depend on the area of vaso-occlusion. Dyspnoea, chest pain, hypertension and proteinuria are all possible symptoms that may signal a sickle-cell crisis, but equally need to be investigated for the more usual pregnancy complications.

Causes may include infection, dehydration, hypotension, hypothermia, hypoxia, acidosis or venous stasis.

Treatment will include the management of any pregnancy complications plus rehydration as necessary, assessment of blood results, appropriate analgesia and an infection screen. A transfusion or exchange transfusion may be needed.

Foetal assessment is necessary and a sickle-cell crisis may lead to an early delivery, although foetal distress during a mother's crisis often disappears as the mother is treated.[38]

Thyroid crisis (storm)

A thyroid crisis may occur in a woman already diagnosed and treated for thyrotoxicosis (hyperthyroidism) or in a woman where the disease has not been diagnosed. It can be caused by failure to take prescribed antithyroid drugs or can be precipitated by stress following infection, trauma or diabetic ketoacidosis.[29] In one study which reported on three maternal deaths, it was suggested that caesarean section for foetal distress was the precipitating factor in two cases, while chest infection was responsible for the other.[39]

Signs and symptoms include extreme pyrexia, tachycardia, congestive cardiac failure, abdominal pain and/or diarrhoea, hypertension, confusion, psychosis and coma. The condition would obviously be suspected more readily if the woman was already known to be diagnosed with thyrotoxicosis.

It is necessary to treat the pyrexia and any infection, as well as treating any cardiac failure and administering specific thyroid therapies.

References

1 Thomas BG (1998) The disempowering concept of risk. *Pract Midwife.* **1** (12): 18–21.

2 Hayashi R (2000) Obstetric collapse. In: LH Kean, PN Baker, DI Edelstone (eds) *Best Practice in Labor Ward Management.* WB Saunders, London.

3 Department of Health (1998) *Why Mothers Die: report on confidential enquiries into maternal deaths in the United Kingdom 1994–1996.* The Stationery Office, London.

4 Deblieux P and Summer W (1996) Acute respiratory failure in pregnancy. *Clin Obstet Gynecol.* **39** (1): 143–52.

5 Mabie W (1996) Critical care obstetrics. In: S Gabbe, J Niebyl and J Simpson (eds) *Obstetrics: normal and problem pregnancies* (3e). Churchill Livingstone, New York.

6 Lewis P and Lanouette J (2000) Principles of critical care. In: W Cohen (ed) *Cherry and Merkatz's Complications of Pregnancy* (5e). Lippincott, Williams & Wilkins, London.

7 Mabie W, Barton J and Sibai B (1992) Adult respiratory distress system in pregnancy. *Am J Obstet Gynecol.* **167** (4:1): 950–7.

8 Hankins G (1997) Acute respiratory distress syndrome. In: S Clark, D Cotton, G Hankins and J Phelan (eds) *Critical Care Obstetrics* (3e). Blackwell Science, Oxford.

9 Moneret-Vautrin D, Beaudouin E, Widmer S et al. (1993) Prospective study of risk factors in natural rubber latex hypersensitivity. *J Allergy Clin Immunol.* **92**: 668–77.

10 Chamberlain G (1991) Abdominal pain in pregnancy. *BMJ.* **302** (6789): 1390–4.

11 Mouad J, Elliott J, Erickson L et al. (2000) Appendicitis in pregnancy: new information that contradicts long-held clinical beliefs. *Am J Obstet Gynecol.* **182** (5): 1027–9.

12 Baskett T (1999) *Essential Management of Obstetric Emergencies* (3e). Clinical Press Limited, Bristol.

13 Abbott J (1999) Emergency management of the obstetric patient. In: G Burrow and

T Duffy (eds) *Medical Complications during Pregnancy* (5e). W B Saunders, Philadelphia.

14 Coleman M and Rund D (1997) Nonobstetric conditions causing hypoxia during pregnancy: asthma and epilepsy. *Am J Obstet Gynecol.* **177** (1): 1–7.

15 Bhatia P and Bhatia K (2000) Pregnancy and the lungs. *Postgrad Med J.* **76** (901): 683–9.

16 Lui S, Wen S, Demissie K et al. (2001) Maternal asthma and pregnancy outcomes: a retrospective cohort study. *Am J Obstet Gynecol.* **184** (2): 90–6.

17 Clarke S, Cotton D, Hawkins G and Phelan J (1997) Severe acute asthma. In: SL Clark (ed) *Critical Care Obstetrics* (3e). Blackwell Science, Massachusetts.

18 Simokle G, Cox S and Cunningham F (1991) Cerebrovascular accident complicating pregnancy and the puerperium. *Obstet Gynecol.* **78** (1): 37–42.

19 Kittner S, Stern B, Feeser B et al. (1996) Pregnancy and the risk of stroke. *NEJM.* **335** (11): 768–74.

20 Sharshar T, Lamy L and Mas J (1995) Incidence and cause of strokes associated with pregnancy and puerperium. *Stroke.* **26**: 930.

21 Donaldson J (1999) Neurological complications. In: G Burrow and T Duffy (eds) *Medical Complications during Pregnancy* (5e). WB Saunders, Philadelphia.

22 Ramin D (1999) Diabetic ketoacidosis in pregnancy. *Obstet Gynecol Clin N Am.* **26** (3): 481–8.

23 Montoro M, Myers V and Mestman J (1993) Out of pregnancy in diabetic ketoacidosis. *Am J Perinatol.* **10**: 17–23.

24 Hagay Z, Weissman A, Lurie S et al. (1994) Reversal of fetal distress following intensive treatment of maternal diabetic ketoacidosis. *Am J Perinatol.* **11**: 430.

25 Jibodu O and Darne F (1997) Spontaneous heterotopic pregnancy presenting with tubal rupture. *Human Repro.* **12**: 1098–9.

26 Ali H (1998) Ectopic pregnancy presenting with obturator nerve pain. *J Accid Emerg Med.* **15**: 192–3.

27 Hajenius P, Mol B, Bossuyt P et al. (2001) Interventions for tubal ectopic pregnancy. In: *The Cochrane Library* (Issue 3). Update Software, Oxford.

28 Paech M, Godkin R and Webster S (1998) Complications of obstetric epidural analgesia and anesthesia: a prospective analysis of 10 995 cases. *Int J Obstet Anesthesia.* **7** (1): 5–11.

29 Cox C and Grady K (1999) *Managing Obstetric Emergencies.* BIOS Scientific Publications, Oxford.

30 Lewis G (ed) (2001) *Why Mothers Die 1997– 1999: The fifth report of the confidential enquiries into maternal deaths in the United Kingdom.* RCOG Press, London.

31 Brown C and Bertolet B (1998) Peripartum cardiomyopathy: a comprehensive review. *Am J Obstet Gynecol.* **178** (2): 409–14.

32 Lampert M, Weinert L, Hibbard J et al. (1997) Contractile reserve in patients with peripartum cardiomyopathy and recovered left ventricular function. *Am J Obstet Gynecol.* **176** (1:1): 189–95.

33 Elkayam U, Tummala P, Rao K et al. (2001) Maternal and fetal outcomes of subsequent pregnancies in women with peripartum cardiomyopathy. *NEJM.* **344** (21): 1567–71.

34 Meller J and Goldman M (2000) Cardiopulmonary disorders. In: W Cohen (ed) *Cherry and Merkatz's Complications of Pregnancy* (5e). Lippincott, Williams & Wilkins, London.

35 Parillo J (1993) Pathogenetic mechanism of septic shock. *NEJM.* **328**: 1471.

36 Clarke S, Cotton D, Hawkins G and Phelan J (1997) Sickle cell crisis. In: SL Clark (ed) *Critical Care Obstetrics* (3e). Blackwell Science, Massachusetts.

37 O'Reilly-Green C (2000) Anaemia. In: W Cohen (ed) *Cherry and Merkatz's Complications of Pregnancy* (5e). Lippincott, Williams & Wilkins, London.

38 Anyaegbunum A, Morel M and Merkatz I (1991) Antepartum fetal surveillance tests during sickle cell crisis. *Am J Obstet Gynecol.* **165** (4:1): 1081–3.

39 Kriplani A, Buckshee K, Bhargava V et al. (1994) Maternal and perinatal outcome in thyrotoxicosis complicating pregnancy. *Eur J Obstet Gynecol Repro Biol.* **54** (3): 159–63.

CHAPTER 12

Assessing and managing risk in midwifery practice

Carol Bates

Introduction

Legislation enables midwives to provide total care during normal pregnancy, childbirth and the postnatal period without recourse to other health professionals. Should there be any deviation from normal, a midwife must call a registered medical practitioner or other health professional who has the skills and experience required to assist her.[1] Consequently traditional midwifery practice, whilst perceiving pregnancy and birth as normal until proved otherwise, has always been mindful of risk.

Historically childbirth was associated with risk and with good reason. Until the turn of the twentieth century, maternal and perinatal mortality and morbidity rates in the western world were high. During the 1920s, the maternal mortality rate was 4.4 deaths per 1000 total births, i.e. 3000 mothers died each year in England and Wales.[2] Women then had frequent pregnancies, often in very poor conditions.[3] Once social conditions improved and the importance of hygiene and nutrition was recognised, childbirth improved for both mother and baby. The introduction of sulphonamide drugs in 1935 and penicillin in 1942 to treat puerperal sepsis resulted in a decrease in maternal mortality by approximately 40–50%.[4] The introduction of ergometrine in the 1930s effectively reduced the number of maternal deaths from postpartum haemorrhage.

Prior to the 1970s, approximately one third of women gave birth at home. Following the publication of the Peel Report,[5] which recommended hospital confinement for all women in the interests of safety, the home birth rate was reduced to approximately 1%.[6] Once the majority of women were giving birth in a hospital environment, this facilitated the application of technology to all aspects of the childbearing process. Towards the end of the twentieth century, routine intervention was commonplace and justified in the interests of obstetric risk management.

Defining risk

A risk management approach to pregnancy and childbirth has prevailed in western society for a number of decades. This was a direct result of the obstetric view that pregnancy and birth could only be considered normal in retrospect. The World Health Organization (WHO) considers that not only has this risk approach to care not been entirely effective because women considered to be low risk have unexpected complications and women considered to be high risk will go on to have an uneventful pregnancy and birth, but that it has also resulted in a disproportionately high number of women finding themselves in a high-risk category.[7]

During the last three decades many risk-scoring systems have been developed. Their purpose is to classify individual women into defined categories for which action can then be planned. O'Leary[8] for example, developed the antenatal risk-scoring system in Table 12.1 for predicting shoulder dystocia.

The problem with such a scoring system is that it clearly categorises women into high, intermediate and negligible risk and this will affect the care they receive. Enkin et al.[9] consider risk-scoring systems should be regarded with caution. They point out that whilst scoring can help to provide a minimum level of care in adequate settings, where provisions are inadequate they can result in a variety of unwarranted interventions and create unnecessary stress and anxiety for women. The WHO considers that the foundation for good decision-making is ongoing assessment of a woman's needs which can change, alongside an ongoing assessment of her birthing potential throughout pregnancy and labour, which can also change.[7]

The label 'high risk' also has cost implications for the National Health Service (NHS) in that it is associated with extra visits, tests and admissions to hospital.[10] Women who are falsely labelled as having pregnancy related complications will at the very least be subjected to further testing and at worst they may suffer unnecessary anxiety and undergo unnecessary and potentially harmful treatment.

Whilst appropriate obstetric intervention has led to improved perinatal outcomes (for example, women with cephalopelvic disproportion or genuine uterine dystocia in labour), regarding all women as being at risk – be it low or high – until they have delivered and proved otherwise has resulted in increasing intervention and soaring caesarean section rates, which in turn increase the risk for mother and baby.

The increasing complexity of the risk approach to childbearing has also had considerable impact upon midwifery practice. It has blurred the boundaries of normality in midwifery practice and whilst the midwife supports women in pregnancy and childbirth regardless of complications developing, a fundamental issue for midwives is the professional autonomy associated with normal birth. Gould[11] argued that midwives have failed to define normality because doctors have so closely defined abnormality and this has allowed the ensuing increasing medicalisation of what should be a normal physiological process for the majority of women.

The Audit Commission Report[12] was the first publication to acknowledge that pregnancy deemed normal only in retrospect produces a very different underlying rationale for the organisation of the maternity services, rather than if pregnancy were perceived as normal until it is proved otherwise. The report also acknowledged that whilst safety must always be of prime concern, the type of maternity care that women receive should reflect that the population is now predominantly healthy and that therefore the nature of the service should be to provide care and support through 'a normal life event'.

The publication of a report such as this, following hard on the heels of *Changing Childbirth*[13] offered genuine opportunities for change in the organisation of the maternity services. The real significance of these reports was that, despite increasing costly litigation in the area of obstetrics, they recommended giving women more choice in their care even though some obstetricians were expressing concern that this would compromise safety for mothers and babies.[14]

Place of birth

The publication of *Changing Childbirth*[13] enabled women to begin to have greater choice in relation

Table 12.1: Antenatal risk-scoring system for shoulder dystocia[8]

Numerical Factor	0	1	2
Estimated foetal weight	4.31 kg	3.86–4.31 kg	3.86 kg
Maternal weight	> 82 kg	68–82 kg	68 kg
Maternal weight gain in pregnancy	> 16 kg	11–16 kg	11 kg
Glucose intolerance	Yes	Suspect	No
Gestational age	> 42 weeks	41–42 weeks	< 41 weeks

A combined score of 0–3 represents great risk, 4–7 intermediate risk and 8–10 negligible risk.

to the place of delivery. Whilst the majority of women continued to give birth in hospital, a small but significant number of women began requesting home births. The numbers of home births continue to rise in certain areas of the UK. A recent investigation into the provision of maternity services gives an average home birth rate in Scotland of 0.4%, Northern Ireland 0.1%, and England and Wales 2%. The provision in England and Wales is very sporadic and the highest home birth rates seem to be in England (for example, in Torquay the home birth rate is 9.7%, Brighton 8%, King's College Hospital in London 6.7%, Stevenage 4.5%). Further statistics on home birth and much more information about all aspects of maternity care provision can be found in the *Good Birth Guide* on the www.drfoster.co.uk website.

As hospital confinement has become the norm, many health professionals view home births as putting the lives of mothers and babies at unnecessary risk. This view is understandable because the medical model of pregnancy and birth that has prevailed for nearly 30 years starts from the premise that childbearing can only be deemed normal in retrospect. However increasing numbers of women are no longer prepared to go along with this view and are requesting home births. The philosophy in *Changing Childbirth*[13] of giving women choice and the forthcoming changes in the provision of healthcare (i.e. primary care) require midwives to revisit risk assessment and management in relation to home birth.

The *Confidential Enquiry into Stillbirths and Deaths in Infancy* (CESDI)[15] conducted a review of 22 cases of planned home births which were associated with the death of the baby. Their findings highlight the need for effective risk assessment and management, expert midwifery skills, good communication skills and efficient emergency support services for those women choosing to give birth at home.

As part of an effective risk management strategy, midwives should ensure that they have the skills required to attend a home birth. They need expert clinical skills in relation to the diagnosis of the onset of labour and monitoring the progress of labour. They should also be trained and competent in maternal and neonatal resuscitation. Midwives should carry the equipment that enables them to do this effectively (*see* Chapter 2).

Midwives should also be aware of what emergency services are available, any guidelines or protocols related to calling them and the average transfer time to hospital. The trend for nearly exclusive hospital delivery over a number of years has resulted in a major reduction in the number of obstetric emergency teams (flying squads). CESDI[15] highlighted what were termed 'transport issues' such as undue delay in response times (more than 1 hour). When making a decision regarding the possible need for transfer to hospital, the midwife needs to consider that it may be appropriate to call for assistance sooner rather than later if the mother lives in a remote area or if it is likely the ambulance may get caught up in heavy traffic.

Making informed choices

Women now have access to a great deal of information from a variety of sources, including the internet. One website www.BirthChoiceUK.com, launched in 2001, is aimed primarily at helping pregnant women to choose where to give birth. The website contains a checklist which guides women through the decision-making process, gives them information about their local options and Department of Health maternity statistics. Many women are no longer prepared to make a choice purely in the light of the information they are given by the midwife or the obstetrician.

It is essential that health professionals do not give information based on their own often irrational fears. Risk assessment and management should be an ongoing process throughout pregnancy. A home birth is an option for fit, healthy women who have uncomplicated pregnancies. If ongoing risk assessment and management is taking place, a woman can be informed of any clinical indications that require her to reconsider her plans for a home birth.

The Department of Health[16] is also of the view that giving and obtaining consent is usually a process rather than a one-off event. Rarely will a woman put her own life and/or that of her baby at risk. A competent pregnant woman may legally refuse any treatment, even if this would be detrimental to the foetus, but the law tends to look at informed consent in isolation. If a pregnant woman has a good relationship with her midwife and trusts her professional judgement, she is unlikely to refuse to listen to any advice or refuse consent to any treatment recommended by the midwife.

Litigation

Most litigation in obstetrics concerns cerebral palsy, a condition that develops in two to three babies in every 1000 live births.[17] The causes of the several different kinds of cerebral palsy remain unknown and it is a highly controversial issue. It has been assumed for many years that perinatal asphyxia was a cause, but recent studies have shown that cerebral palsy is more often associated with prematurity, infection, intrauterine growth restriction, congenital abnormalities and multiple pregnancy.[18]

What is interesting is that despite a marked fall in perinatal mortality rates, the cerebral palsy rate has remained virtually unchanged, that is two to three in every 1000 live births since data began to be analysed in 1956.[19] The medical profession would like to clearly define the clinical differences between cerebral palsy caused by hypoxia in complicated pregnancies and cerebral palsy as a direct result of hypoxia during labour and birth.

In 1997, an International Cerebral Palsy Taskforce was set up to carry out an extensive review of all literature relating to cerebral palsy. Their findings were published as an international consensus statement. The conclusion of the taskforce was that recent research suggested that the causes of a large majority of cerebral palsies are multifactorial and due to mostly unpreventable events during either foetal development or the neonatal period.[20]

The purpose of the statement was to help both health professionals and courts of law, but it has yet to make an impact on the legal profession, and litigation for cerebral palsy and other birth injuries continues to cost the NHS huge sums of money. In 1990 the legal aid rules were revised and from thereon all claims on behalf of infants became state funded.[21] This resulted in an increase in the number of claims and litigation costs have escalated. Risk financing became an urgent problem for the NHS and resulted in the setting up of the National Health Service Litigation Authority (NHSLA) to formally address issues surrounding the assessment, management and financing of risk.

The National Health Service Litigation Authority

The London-based NHSLA has introduced risk management strategies for care throughout the NHS and most trusts now participate in the Clinical Negligence Scheme for Trusts (CNST). Trusts contribute to the scheme and their contributions are set against the clinical risk management standards[22] set out in the scheme. Standard 12 relates to management and communication in maternity care (see Table 12.2). It is very broad based and acknowledges the multidisciplinary nature of maternity care and the need for good communication between health professionals. The need for regularly updated evidence-based policies to manage what are described as key conditions or situations on the labour ward is highlighted.

Standard 12 is about good practice which includes good clinical and decision-making skills, keeping up to date through continuing professional development, communication, documentation and record-keeping, and a clear line of referral in the event of problems occurring.

Many of the key conditions are familiar to all midwives. For example, women with diabetes, severe hypertension and major haemoglobinopathy require specific care, as do those where prostaglandins and antibiotics are proposed. Medical or obstetric management is the only appropriate course, and care and product use should be based on evidence-based guidelines.

Emergency management of most of the key situations, for example eclampsia, uterine rupture, shoulder dystocia and severe postpartum haemorrhage, comes within the scope of midwifery practice; other situations such as failed adult intubation do not. With appropriate monitoring and care during pregnancy and labour, these situations may possibly be avoided and traditionally they are situations of which midwives have always been mindful and have tried to avoid. Whilst all health care professionals should be able to manage emergencies effectively, risk assessment and management should be such that these emergencies are at least reduced and at best avoided wherever possible.

Apart from waterbirth, the main focus of Standard 12 is the management of abnormality and emergencies. It is worthwhile remembering that the majority of women are fit and healthy and have uncomplicated pregnancies. Obstetric emergencies are relatively rare but they require prompt diagnosis and treatment and all midwives should be aware of the signs and symptoms. Midwives should also take part in regular multidisciplinary emergency drills to ensure they can respond efficiently and effectively.[23]

Table 12.2: Standard 12: Management and communication in maternity care

Standard 12	Management and Communication in Maternity Care
12.1.1	The arrangements are clear concerning which professional is responsible for the patient's care at all times.
12.1.2	There are referenced, evidence-based multidisciplinary policies for the management of all key conditions/situations on the labour ward. These are subject to review at intervals of not more than three years.
12.1.2.1	Anatomical definition and repair of third degree perineal tear.
12.1.2.2	Antepartum haemorrhage including placental abruption.
12.1.2.3	Breech presentation including version and selection for vaginal delivery.
12.1.2.4	Diabetes.
12.1.2.5	Eclampsia.
12.1.2.6	Failed adult intubation (may be in anaesthetic policy).
12.1.2.7	Major haemoglobinopathy.
12.1.2.8	Management of women who decline blood products.
12.1.2.9	Multiple pregnancy.
12.1.2.10	Prolapsed cord.
12.1.2.11	Prophylactic antibiotics for caesarean section.
12.1.2.12	Prostaglandins use.
12.1.2.13	Rupture of uterus.
12.1.2.14	Severe hypertension.
12.1.2.15	Severe postpartum haemorrhage.
12.1.2.16	Shoulder dystocia.
12.1.2.17	Thromboprophylaxis in caesarean section.
12.1.2.18	Unexplained intrapartum/postpartum collapse including amniotic fluid embolism.
12.1.2.19	Waterbirth.
12.1.3	There is an agreed mechanism for direct referral to a consultant from a midwife.
12.1.4	There is a personal handover of care when medical or midwifery shifts change.
12.1.5	There is a clear documented system for management and communication throughout the key stages of maternity care.
12.1.6	All clinicians should attend six-monthly multidisciplinary in-service education/training sessions on the management of 'high risk' labours and CTG interpretations.
12.2.1	There is a lead consultant obstetrician and clinical midwife manager.
12.2.2	Consultant supervision should be available for the labour ward for a minimum of 40 hours per week of scheduled sessions.
12.3.1	Emergency caesarean section can be undertaken rapidly and within a short enough period to eliminate unacceptable delay. The delivery interval in caesarean section for foetal distress is subject to an annual audited standard.
12.3.2	There is a personal handover to obstetric locums, either by post-holder, or a senior member of the team and vice versa.

Printed with the permission of the NHSLA.[22]

An under-reported issue in risk management is the maternal morbidity rate. An investigation of long-term health problems directly associated with childbirth carried out in Birmingham revealed that of 11 701 women surveyed, 47% suffered ill health after childbirth. The problems reported included depression, anxiety, chronic backache, headaches, migraine, paraesthesia and stress incontinence. For many women these problems were still present nine years after giving birth.[24] It has also been recognised that routine obstetric intervention has created psychological and physiological problems that profoundly affect the lives of women for many years afterwards.[25]

Planned reforms for clinical negligence

Despite the work of the NHSLA and the efforts of trusts to develop effective risk management strategies, a report published by the National Audit Office[26] confirms that the cost of litigation continues to soar in England. According to this report the NHS must make provision of at least £4 billion for claims already put forward and for those known to be in the pipeline. The report also highlights the length of time it takes to settle a claim, which is around five years. This is too long for patients generally and certainly too long for parents of a handicapped child.

In July 2001 the Secretary of State for Health announced plans to publish a White Paper in 2002 setting out reforms to the system dealing with clinical negligence claims. He agreed the present system was too slow and bureaucratic. The Chief Medical Officer is to chair a committee to look at suggestions to make the system faster and fairer for both patients and health professionals. The key issues to be addressed will be mediation rather than litigation, and no-fault liability. This will mean the claimant does not have to prove who, if anyone, was at fault. There would be fixed tariff payments related to the type of injury and settlements, with parents receiving regular payments rather than a lump sum.

The Government is clearly being very pragmatic about clinical negligence. It is accepting that, with the best of intentions, some accidents will still occur and therefore avoidable harm to users of the service will continue. What is important is that midwives have greater input into the development of standards of maternity care and the Government must acknowledge the professional responsibilities carried by midwives often under very difficult conditions.

The NHS modernisation programme

Clinical governance in the interests of reducing litigation costs and promoting patient safety is integral to the Government's modernisation programme, which is being carried forward by the NHS Modernisation Agency based in Leicester. The agency provides a Clinical Governance Support Team (CGST) established in 1999 to support the implementation of clinical governance. One of their programmes which is of vital importance to midwives is *Delivering Healthy Babies*. It began in July 2001 and will continue until September 2002. The Agency believes this clinically focused,

multiprofessional programme will achieve improvements in maternity care by enabling health professionals to challenge outdated roles and practices and increase efficiency and safety at a local level. Visit their website www.cgsupport.org for more information.

Midwifery aspects to assessment and management of risk

The care women receive during pregnancy and birth has become complex. Whilst it requires the collaboration of an increasing number of health professionals, the midwife remains at the centre of this care. As this chapter has already shown, there is a tremendous political interest in the functioning of the NHS and the outcome of care, especially in relation to risk management and clinical negligence. The Government intends that its multifactorial clinical governance programme will exercise control over all aspects of patient care in order to improve the outcome of care and at the same time control the escalating costs of the NHS. The National Institute for Clinical Excellence (NICE) for example, requires research based evidence on both therapeutic and cost effectiveness of drugs before they can be prescribed and produces numerous evidence-based guidelines for health professionals.

Expert midwifery practice supports and enhances the physiological processes of childbearing. This should be fundamental to any risk management strategy for pregnant women. The remainder of this chapter will broadly discuss aspects of midwifery practice that lend themselves naturally to risk assessment and management.

Antenatal care

A fundamental component of antenatal care is to identify those pregnancies that are at greater than average risk. This process begins with the antenatal booking visit. Whether the booking visit takes place at hospital, local health centre or in the woman's home, it provides the midwife with an opportunity to initiate a positive relationship with the woman and lay a firm foundation on which to build during the rest of the pregnancy.[27,28]

A study carried out by Methven[29] found that the focus of the booking visit was on taking an obstetric history at the expense of developing a relationship with a woman. It was this kind of impersonal care that led women to campaign for changes in the organisation of the maternity services and culminated in the publication of the *Changing Childbirth* report.[13]

The midwife's ability to communicate effectively but in a friendly, professional manner is of vital importance at this visit. For the communication to be entirely effective, there should be a two-way interaction between the woman and the midwife. As well as gaining information about a woman's family, medical and obstetric history, the booking visit should enable the midwife to assess a woman's social, emotional and psychological needs as well as her physical condition.

Observation skills

Effective risk assessment also requires good skills of observation. When meeting a woman for the first time, the midwife should take note of her physical appearance. All midwives are familiar with the potential significance of short stature and will notice if a woman has a physical defect that may interfere with the normal processes of childbearing or if she is under- or over-nourished. However, of equal importance is observing a woman's psychological well-being. Not all women look forward to motherhood.

Pregnancy is a time of inner turmoil and self re-appraisal for women.[30] The roots of postnatal depression, which continues to affect one in ten women, can often be found in pregnancy and before. It could be argued that the biomedical emphasis of antenatal care has resulted in greater importance being placed upon the physical well-being of mother and foetus, as well as preparation for labour and birth, at the expense of emotional preparation for the role transition and parenting. Observational skills enable a more holistic approach to risk assessment and management and should be employed throughout pregnancy, labour and birth.

History taking

If the history taking is to be beneficial to both mother and midwife, it must not be rushed. The midwife must also make adjustments as necessary to meet individual women's needs. For example an interpreter must be present for those women who do not speak English or working women may prefer an evening visit at home, as might a woman who already has young children. Sometimes a partner or other members of the family may be present and the midwife should be sensitive to the fact that there may be information that the woman will not give in the presence of others. All women should be given an opportunity to speak with the midwife when they are alone.

Social and health inequalities

Social disadvantage has an enormous impact on childbearing. It often goes hand in hand with health inequalities, which increase the risk of perinatal morbidity and mortality, for example in the birth of low birth weight babies. The Winterton report[31] highlighted the importance of the social context of childbearing and health inequalities and expressed the view that the outcome of pregnancy was dependent to a large degree on a woman's social environment. A study conducted by Oakley et al.[32] confirmed this view, while also highlighting the importance of both social and midwifery support.

When assisting women to make choices regarding the care they are to receive, the midwife should always take into consideration a woman's social situation. Some women may be caught in a poverty trap, possibly coping with difficult living conditions or even homelessness. Any advice a midwife gives should be based on the reality of a woman's life. This view is supported by the findings of a longitudinal study carried out in Liverpool to discover how women felt about information that was provided regarding pregnancy, labour and parenthood. The results of the study demonstrated that for information to be meaningful to women it had to be tailored to meet individual needs.[33]

Medical history

As the Audit Commission[12] pointed out the population is now predominantly healthy and maternity care should reflect this. However, midwives still need to inquire about any physical, psychiatric or psychological illness, operations or accidents that could complicate pregnancy or birth. A woman's family history is also important and many women now welcome the opportunity for prenatal diagnosis. Equally there are those women for whom it is inappropriate and their wishes should be respected.

It is also important to explore the need to screen for infection. The NHS Executive has published guidelines on both hepatitis B and HIV testing in pregnancy.[34,35] The Department of Health supported by The Royal College of Midwives has also produced information leaflets for midwives on both hepatitis B and HIV testing in pregnancy.[36,37]

Midwives should also be aware of the implications of maternal Group B Streptococcus (GBS) infection in pregnancy. GBS is a leading cause of early onset neonatal sepsis.[38] It is transmitted to the neonate during birth. Mothers may be chronic, intermittent or transient carriers of GBS and therefore the detection rates during pregnancy vary. The Public Health Laboratory Service (PHLS) recently published *Interim good practice recommendations for the prevention of early-onset neonatal Group B Streptococcus infection in the UK* on its website. See the website at http://www/phls.org.uk/advice/goodpracticeStrepto.pdf for more information.

Previous pregnancies and births

Details of all previous pregnancies, labours and puerperia are essential. A woman's previous experiences of pregnancy and birth may have implications for the present pregnancy and the type of care she should receive. They may also have implications for place of birth. For example, a woman may give a history of a previous large baby and a birth complicated by shoulder dystocia. However it should not mean that a woman be put into a high- or low-risk category at the outset. There should be an ongoing assessment throughout pregnancy and labour.

Whilst acknowledging that shoulder dystocia can occur unexpectedly, O'Leary[8] still considered that the best approach to shoulder dystocia was prevention. He suggested that there was a need for a high level of 'intuition and anticipatory knowledge' to avoid what he described as a potentially 'catastrophic event' (*see* Chapter 9 for further information on shoulder dystocia).

This degree of vigilance and anticipation means the midwife will not be caught unawares if shoulder dystocia does occur. If the midwife has also kept up to date with emergency practice drills, she will demonstrate the ability to both assess and manage clinical risk. It is important that midwives and other health professionals practice emergency drills as part of their continuing professional development to enable them to take prompt, appropriate action. This is in keeping with the philosophy of the NHSLA Standard 12.

The above approach to risk assessment and management can be applied to all aspects of antenatal care. It enables the midwife to be pro-active rather than reactive, anticipating problems that may occur, rather than managing them when they do. It also promotes holistic woman-centred care by meeting women's psychological as well as physical needs and encourages them to be part of the decision-making process. This will give women a sense of being in control of the child-bearing process. It also promotes the clinical expertise of the midwife and supports a multi-disciplinary approach to care.

Assessing and managing risk in labour

Whilst care in labour has become increasingly medicalised and many interventions such as amniotomy, electronic foetal monitoring and epidural analgesia have become commonplace, certain midwifery practices continue to be fundamental to risk assessment and management.

Abdominal examination

A wealth of information can be gained from an abdominal examination. Abdominal palpation enables the midwife to assess foetal size, and define the position of the foetus and the degree of engagement of the presentation. Foetal movements can be observed; excessive foetal movement can be associated with hypoxia.

Abdominal examination should include regular assessment of the bladder because the sensation of wanting to empty the bladder is diminished during labour and the use of epidural analgesia results in women having no sensation of wanting to pass urine. It is well documented that a full bladder may delay the progress of labour by impeding descent of the presenting part. This will in turn inhibit good uterine contractions and efficient dilatation of the cervix. A full bladder during the third stage of labour has the potential to interfere with uterine muscle retraction and the process of placental separation causing a postpartum haemorrhage.

Regular abdominal palpation throughout the first and second stage of labour enables the midwife to monitor the descent of the foetal head through the pelvis and is a very useful risk assessment and management tool.

Urinalysis is also useful as part of the clinical assessment process. Maternal ketoacidosis inhibits uterine contractions and predisposes to maternal and foetal distress and possibly postpartum haemorrhage.

Monitoring uterine contractions

The length, strength and frequency of uterine contractions should be palpated on a regular basis because the nature of contractions changes throughout labour. The midwife needs to be vigilant and observe whether uterine action is co-ordinate or inco-ordinate as this has implications for both mother and baby and may affect women's choices in relation to the management of their labour. If oxytocin is being used to either induce or augment labour, the midwife needs to be particularly vigilant when monitoring uterine action.

Vaginal examination

In the interests of risk assessment and management, it is essential that a vaginal examination is always preceded by an abdominal palpation. The combination of external and internal findings gives the skilled midwife a mental picture of the progress of labour.[39] Midwives should be wary when estimating the level or position of the presenting part in relation to the ischial spines as moulding of the foetal skull or the presence of caput succedaneum can result in the presenting part appearing to be lower than it really is. Abdominal palpation is the only reliable method of monitoring descent of the foetal head through the pelvis.

The findings on vaginal examination tend to be subjective, with different health professionals disagreeing about the level of the presenting part or the dilatation of the cervix. For this reason it is advisable that the same person carries out all vaginal examinations on a particular woman.

Listening to the foetal heart

The foetal heart should be assessed on completion of an abdominal or vaginal examination. It can be carried out using either a Pinard's stethoscope or Doppler ultrasound apparatus (Doptone or Sonicaid) and the foetal heart rate and rhythm should be noted.

If intermittent monitoring is being used MacDonald[40] recommends that the foetal heart is listened to for one minute at the following intervals to enable the midwife to hear any variations:

- every 15 minutes during the first stage of labour

- after every contraction towards the end of the first stage of labour

- after every contraction throughout the second stage.

When using intermittant monitoring if any foetal heart rate abnormality occurs, electronic foetal heart rate monitoring should be used to assess and clarify the situation. Foetal blood sampling may be necessary, and even if this is within normal limits, electronic foetal heart monitoring should be considered for the rest of the labour.

More recently NICE published guidelines on the use of electronic foetal monitoring.[41] The guidelines acknowledge that current evidence does not support the use of an admission cardiotocography (CTG) and therefore they do not recommend its use in low-risk women. NICE also supports intermittent auscultation in labour for women who are healthy and have had an uncomplicated pregnancy, reflecting similar recommendations made earlier by MacDonald.[40] In the active phase of labour the foetal heart should be listened to after a contraction for at least a full minute at the following stages:

- every 15 minutes in the first stage of labour

- every 5 minutes in the second stage of labour.

Continuous electronic foetal monitoring (EFM) should be offered on the following bases:

- if there is evidence on auscultation of a baseline less than 110 or greater than 160 bpm

- if there is evidence on auscultation of any decelerations

- if any intrapartum risk factors, as described in the local clinical practice algorithm, develop.

Spiby[42] highlighted the difficulties that such guidelines can present for midwifery practice. She says midwives are expressing concern about not doing an admission CTG because it has become a routine component of care and apparently gives them reassurance at the beginning of labour. Midwives are also concerned about the views of obstetricians and risk managers on this issue. They too are expressing concern about the risk management implications of not carrying out an admission trace and as Spiby points out, midwives do not work in isolation. There is also the belief that intermittent auscultation during the first stage of labour will be difficult to achieve in practice, although no reason is given for this view, and during the second stage of labour women will find it too intrusive.

These views demonstrate the power of technology, how it can so easily replace midwifery practice skills and the blind belief that technology is fundamental to risk assessment and management. When EFM was introduced in the 1960s, there was a high expectation that it would allow early recognition of hypoxia and thereby enable timely intervention to avoid death or brain damage in the newborn. However, in the mid-1990s a Cochrane review[43] of evidence from randomised controlled trials concluded that the only benefit of EFM was a reduction in neonatal seizures and, unless EFM was used in conjunction with foetal blood sampling, it was associated with an increase in caesarean section rates. In addition EFM has not reduced perinatal mortality rates and as mentioned above cerebral palsy rates have remained the same since the 1950s.

Mary Macintosh, Director of the *Confidential Enquiry into Stillbirths and Deaths in Infancy*, considers there is a conflict between the findings of the annual CESDI reports and the results of randomised trials on EFM. She offers an interesting critique of the strengths and weaknesses of EFM research methodology and highlights the difficulties in relation to research in this area. She remains of the view that the conflict she describes is unlikely to be resolved.[44]

Enkin et al.[45] have been promoting effective care in pregnancy and birth since 1989. To be effective, care must be evidence-based. This sounds very straightforward but often data is considered to be of insufficient and inadequate quality and therefore should not be used as a basis for recommending a change in practice. The admission trace is a good example of this and yet the practice has become commonplace and according to Spiby, continues. It could also be argued that the admission trace has the potential to give midwives a sense of false security. Much depends upon the interpretation of the CTG. Technology, whilst a useful tool, can never replace the skills of the competent, professional midwife.

Second stage of labour

This stage is said to begin when the cervix is fully dilated. However, it is often not known exactly when the cervix becomes fully dilated and full dilatation may not coincide with a woman's urge to bear down. Women who have epidural analgesia may find the urge to push is reduced or delayed or they may not experience the feeling at all.

The second stage of labour has long been considered to be a time of special risk for the foetus and it was probably this fear that triggered the invention of forceps to expedite delivery. Lagercrantz and Slotkin[46] however insist that the stress of 'journeying through the birth canal' is not harmful to most infants. The evidence they have gathered over a period of twenty years convinces them that the foetus is well equipped to withstand the stress of being born. They cite the physiological surge of foetal catecholamines that occurs during labour as being both a protective mechanism and essential to the neonate's survival outside of the womb.[46]

The key risk management factors for midwifery practice in the second stage of labour are identified below.

Active pushing

There have been many studies comparing different approaches to pushing. Active pushing has often been encouraged to ensure women deliver within a prescribed time limit dependent upon parity. A national survey in England during the 1980s found that there was a time limit of one hour for primigravidae and thirty minutes for multigravidae.[47] According to Sleep[48] in studies of deliveries where sustained or early bearing down was encouraged, there was a predisposition to abnormalities of the foetal heart rate and low Apgar scores. The midwife should consider not promoting active pushing until the presenting part is visible at the vulva.

Length of the second stage of labour

A prolonged second stage of labour has been statistically associated with poor foetal outcome including neonatal seizures.[49] However Sleep[48] considers these associations are not sufficient justification for concluding that the length of the second stage *per se* is the root cause of poor foetal outcome. She concluded that if maternal and foetal condition is satisfactory and there is evidence of steady progress, there are no grounds for intervention. What is important is that the midwife carefully monitors descent of the presenting part during the second stage and does not instil a sense of urgency into a woman. This will create unnecessary anxiety and interfere with normal physiological processes.[50]

The timing of an episiotomy

Assessing the need for an episiotomy and the timing of its execution need to be just right. If it is carried out too soon it may be too small and extend during delivery, and there is also the risk of haemorrhage from the incision.

Difficulties with delivery of the shoulders

Mortimore and McNabb[51] carried out a six-year retrospective analysis of shoulder dystocia and they suggest that spontaneous birth of the shoulders may be hindered by the woman's position. For example, adoption of a semi-recumbent position will put pressure on the sacrum, which effectively reduces the anteroposterior diameter of the pelvic outlet. They also support the view that epidural analgesia may retard or eliminate both descent and rotation of the shoulders. There is also the possibility of unnecessary haste with some midwives not waiting for internal rotation of the

shoulders. Attempting delivery before internal rotation has occurred may give the impression that the shoulders are stuck when in fact they are not, but have just not rotated into the widest diameter of the pelvic outlet.

Third stage of labour

This stage is considered to be a hazardous time for women with the attendant potential for postpartum haemorrhage, retained placenta and very rarely, an inverted uterus (*see* Chapter 8). There is much the midwife can do to avoid these complications (*see* Chapter 10). Inappropriate manipulation of the uterus, commonly called 'fundal fiddling', remains a common cause of incomplete placental separation.[52]

Active management of the third stage of labour has become commonplace. The routine prophylactic administration of oxytoxic drugs has been criticised, but a large number of studies have now taken place and the results suggest that routine administration of oxytoxics will reduce the risk of postpartum haemorrhage.[45]

If a woman declines active management of the third stage of labour, the midwife should explain to her that in the event of a postpartum haemorrhage there would be a need for therapeutic oxytocin. This discussion should be documented in the case notes.

Documentation and record-keeping

Accurate documentation and record-keeping is fundamental to risk assessment and management, while enabling effective communication between health professionals. Rule 42 of the *Midwives Rules and Code of Practice*[53] is specific to record-keeping. It states: 'a practising midwife shall keep as contemporaneously as is reasonable detailed records of observations, care given ...' The *Midwives Rules* are supported by the *Code of Practice,* and while the former is binding on the midwife's practice, the latter is significant in that it is not prescriptive in relation to details of midwifery care. This is because of the comprehensive nature of midwifery education and training and because each midwife is accountable for her own practice. The *Code of Practice* draws attention to Rule 42. It states: 'A midwife's records are an essential aspect of her practice and the midwife's attention is drawn in particular to Rule 42'.

The document *Guidelines for Records and Record Keeping*[54] makes it clear that record-keeping is an essential and integral part of all care given. It goes one step further than previous publications and states, 'good record keeping is a mark of the skilled and safe practitioner'.

The guidelines also remind health professionals that they should assume that any entries made in the case notes will be scrutinised by others at some point. Consequently records must be accurate, current and comprehensive. They should be legible, indelible, clear and unambiguous. Abbreviations and acronyms should not be used. All records should be timed and signed by the person making them. They should also be contemporaneous and demonstrate the chronology of events, documenting observations, decisions, interventions and outcomes of all care given.

The fourth CESDI[55] made criticisms about the poor quality of record-keeping and drew attention to the consequences of poor communication between different health professionals. These sentiments were echoed in the most recent CESDI[56] with particular emphasis on poor documentation. Bryne[57] considers that the issue of poor record-keeping by healthcare professionals is a recurrent one. She highlights the need for developing criteria for good record-keeping and suggests multidisciplinary workshops where all members of the health care team are required to read each others' documentation and record-keeping. This would be an innovative way of updating and maintaining standards of record-keeping.

The clinical environment

The concept that each midwife is responsible and accountable for her own practice[53] has encouraged an individualised approach to risk management through the supervision of midwives rather than a more systematic approach. This approach has its drawbacks in that individual midwives may feel they are being targeted which can lead to a climate of fear that is not helpful to effective clinical risk assessment and management.

A more systematic approach to risk management has been primarily obstetric led and

this has resulted in maternity units and especially labour wards becoming permeated with an interventionist approach to care in the name of risk management. This process has to some extent marginalised midwifery practice and resulted in routine practices, many of which are not evidence-based (for example, a time limit on the duration of the second stage of labour), which have not been in the best interests of either women or the midwifery profession.

Quilliam[58] suggests that while the modern discourse of risk management may be unfamiliar to midwives, the concept is not. She argues that midwives have always been taught to recognise abnormalities that require referral and are able to deal with life-threatening emergencies that require taking decisive action. Quilliam does not support the obstetric view that pregnancy can only be normal in retrospect but she points out that if midwives actively embrace clinical risk management they will ensure that maternity services are both safe and woman-centred.

The success or otherwise of midwifery clinical risk assessment and management will depend to a large extent upon the clinical environment in which midwives work. Kirkham[59] conducted a study of the culture of midwifery in the NHS in England and her findings reveal that the traditional midwifery activities of support and care continue but within organisations with very different values. Kirkham describes the voice of midwifery as being muted and midwives as being in a 'professional state of learned helplessness and guilt'.

The medicalisation of childbearing, NHS management practices, the rise of clinical negligence claims and the fear this engenders have all had a part to play in bringing about this state of affairs. Since the 1970s midwives have accommodated many changes within the organisation of the maternity services that have profoundly affected the way they work, and they have embraced and supported obstetric practices, which have effectively marginalised midwifery practice. It is therefore understandable that Kirkham[59] found so many midwives in a state of 'learned helplessness'. Consequently although organisations such as the National Childbirth Trust and the Association for Improvements in Maternity Services are calling upon midwives to empower women, they cannot do this effectively until they have experienced empowerment themselves.

Conclusion

Risk assessment and management will remain high on the Government's agenda even if there are reforms to the system. However, the stage is set for change and midwives should use this opportunity to achieve empowerment for themselves. There are already systems in place that are potentially supportive and protective of midwifery practice; for example, supervision of midwives. Used appropriately, these systems are excellent risk assessment and management tools. Kirkham[60] recommends that we also need to foster mutual support among midwives and build a network of supportive colleagues as further excellent risk management strategies.

The midwifery profession has relatively small numbers, who have always networked effectively at a local, national and international level. This networking was greatly assisted by the statutory requirement for all midwives to attend a five-day refresher course every five years. Such courses gathered midwives from throughout the UK and abroad. The implementation of the Post Registration Education and Practice (PREP) project has gradually changed this practice and this opportunity for networking has been lost. We must now look for new ways of effective networking, such as visiting midwifery websites and chat rooms, attending study days and conferences and at a local level, organising midwifery practice groups to discuss and debate all aspects of midwifery care.

If midwives have a strong sense of professional identity, this will make the profession strong. Strong midwives are motivated to learn for enhanced competence and become expert clinical practitioners, supporting and enhancing the physiological processes of childbearing, using interventions appropriately, able to manage abnormality and deal promptly and efficiently with emergencies. This is effective risk management. Strong midwives also have the potential to become strong leaders. Leadership is about setting direction for others, challenging the *status quo* and opening up possibilities that enable both personal and professional development: factors fundamental to successful midwifery risk assessment and management.

References

1 United Kingdom Central Council for Nursing, Midwifery and Health Visiting (1998) *Midwives Rules and Code of Practice.* UKCC, London.

2 The Royal College of Midwives (2000) *Reassessing Risk: a midwifery perspective.* Royal College of Midwives, London.

3 Lewis J (1990) Mothers and maternity politics in the 20th century. In: J Garcia, R Kilpatrick and M Richards (eds) *The Politics of Maternity Care.* Clarendon Press, Oxford.

4 Tew M (1998) *Safer Childbirth?: a critical history of maternity care* (3e). Free Association Books, London.

5 Department of Health and Social Security Standing Maternity and Midwifery Advisory Committee (1970) (Chairman J Peel) *Domiciliary Midwifery and Maternity Bed Needs.* HMSO, London.

6 Campbell R and Macfarlane A (1994) *Where to be born?: the debate and the evidence* (2e). National Perinatal Epidemiology Unit, Oxford.

7 World Health Organization (1999) *Care in Normal Birth: a practical guide.* World Health Organization, Geneva.

8 O'Leary JA (1992) *Shoulder Dystocia and Birth Injury: prevention and treatment.* McGraw-Hill, New York.

9 Enkin M, Keirse M and Chalmers I (1989) *Effective Care in Pregnancy and Childbirth.* Oxford University Press, Oxford.

10 Savage W (1986) Changing attitudes to intervention: is it possible to reverse the rise in the number of caesareans? *Nurs Times Nurs Mirror.* **82** (22): 63–4.

11 Gould D (2000) Normal Labour: a concept analysis. *J Adv Nurs.* **31** (2): 418–27.

12 Audit Commission (1997) *First Class Delivery Service: improving maternity services in England and Wales.* Audit Commission Publications, London.

13 Department of Health (1993) *Changing Childbirth Part 1: report of the expert maternity group.* HMSO, London.

14 Drife J (1995) Reducing risk in obstetrics. In: C Vincent (ed) *Clinical Risk Management.* BMJ Publishing Group, London.

15 Maternal and Child Health Research Consortium (1998) *Confidential Enquiry into Stillbirths and Deaths in Infancy* (Fifth Annual Report). CESDI, London.

16 Department of Health (2001) *12 Key Points on Consent: the law in England.* The Stationery Office, London.

17 Bakketeig LS (1999) Only a minor part of cerebral palsy cases begin in labour. *BMJ.* **319**: 1016–17.

18 Floyd L (2000) Acute intrapartum events and cerebral palsy: an international consensus statement (a summary). *Pract Midwife.* **3** (2): 32–3.

19 Bryce R, Stanley F and Blair E (1989) The effects of intrapartum care on the risk of impairments in childhood. In: I Chalmers, M Enkin and MJ Keirse (eds) *Effective Care in Pregnancy and Childbirth* (Vol 1). Oxford University Press, Oxford.

20 MacLennan A (1999) A template for defining a causal relation between acute intrapartum events and cerebral palsy: international consensus statement. *BMJ.* **319**: 1054–9.

21 Capstick B (ed) Mason D and Edwards P (1993) *Litigation: a risk management guide for midwives.* Royal College of Midwives, London.

22 National Health Service Litigation Authority (1999) *Clinical Negligence Scheme for Trusts* Clinical Risk Management Standards. NHSLA, London.

23 McGeown P (2001) Practice recommendations for obstetric emergencies. *Br J Midwif.* **9** (2): 71–3.

24 MacArthur J, Lewis M and Knox EG (1991) *Health after Childbirth.* HMSO, London.

25 Robinson J (1995) Behavioural iatrogenesis. *Br J Midwif.* **3** (6): 335.

26 Comptroller and Auditor General (2001) *Handling clinical negligence claims in England* (Sessions 2000–2001). National Audit Office, London.

27 Reid M and Garcia J (1989) Women's views of antenatal care. In: I Chalmers, M Enkin and MJ Keirse (eds) *Effective Care in Pregnancy and Childbirth* (Vol 1). Oxford University Press, Oxford .

28 Hutton E (1994) What women want from midwives. *Br J Midwif.* **2** (12): 608–11.

29 Methven RC (1982) *The antenatal booking interview: recording an obstetric history or relating with a mother-to-be?* Proceedings of the Research and the Midwife Conference, Glasgow.

30 Raphael-Leff J (1993) *Pregnancy: the inside story.* Sheldon Press, London.

31 House of Commons Select Committee (1992) *Maternity Services* (Sessions 1991–1992; Second Report). HMSO, London.

32 Oakley A, Hickey D and Rajan L (1996) Social support in pregnancy: does it have long-term effects? *J Repro Infant Psychol.* **14**: 7–22.

33 Lavender T, Moffatt H and Rixon S (2000) Do we provide information to women in the best way? *Br J Midwif.* **8** (12): 679–775.

34 NHS Executive (1998) *Screening of Pregnant Women for Hepatitis B and Immunisation of Babies at Risk.* Department of Health, London.

35 NHS Executive (1999) *Reducing Mother to Baby Transmission of HIV.* Department of Health, London.

36 Department of Health (2000) *Hepatitis B Testing in Pregnancy.* Department of Health, London.

37 Department of Health (1998) *HIV Testing in Pregnancy.* Department of Health, London.

38 Fey R, Stuart J and George R (1999) *Neonatal group B streptococcal disease in England and Wales 1981–1997.* Proceedings of the Royal College of Paediatrics and Child Health Spring Meeting, London.

39 Bates C (ed) (2001) *Midwifery Clinical Practice: the first stage of labour.* Royal College of Midwives, London.

40 MacDonald D (1989), cited Cooke P (1992) Fetal monitoring – a questionable practice? *Mod Midwife.* **2** (2): 8–11.

41 National Institute for Clinical Excellence (2001) *The Use of Electronic Fetal Monitoring.* NICE, London.

42 Spiby H (2001) The NICE guidelines on electronic fetal monitoring. *Br J Midwif.* **9** (8): 489.

43 Neilson JP (1995) Electronic fetal monitoring + scalp blood sampling vs. intermittent auscultation in labour. In: *The Cochrane Library* (Issue 2). Update Software, Oxford.

44 Macintosh MCM (2001) Continuous fetal heart rate monitoring: is there a conflict between confidential enquiry findings and results of randomized trials? *J Royal Soc Med.* **94**: 14–16.

45 Enkin E, Keirse MJNC, Neilson J et al. (eds) (2000) *A Guide to Effective Care in Pregnancy and Childbirth* (3e). Oxford University Press, Oxford.

46 Lagercrantz H and Slotkin TA (1986) The 'stress' of being born. *Scient Am.* **254** (4): 100–7.

47 Garcia J, Garforth S and Ayers S (1986) *Midwives confined: labour ward policies and routines.* Proceedings of the Research and the Midwife Conference, 1985, Manchester.

48 Sleep J, Roberts J and Chalmers I (1989) Care during the second stage of labour.

In: I Chalmers, M Enkin and M Keirse (eds) *Effective Care in Pregnancy and Childbirth* (Vol 2). Oxford University Press, Oxford.

49 Minchom P, Niswander K, Chalmers I et al. (1987) Antecedents and outcome of very early neonatal seizures in infants born at or after term. *Br J Obstet Gynaecol.* **94** (5): 431–9.

50 Bates C (ed) (2001) *Midwifery Clinical Practice: the second stage of labour.* Royal College of Midwives, London.

51 Mortimore V and McNabb M (1998) A six-year retrospective analysis of shoulder dystocia and delivery of the shoulders. *Midwifery.* **14** (3): 162–73.

52 McDonald S (1999) Physiology and Management of the Third Stage of Labour. In: VR Bennett and LK Brown (eds) *Myles Textbook for Midwives.* Churchill Livingstone, Edinburgh.

53 United Kingdom Central Council for Nursing, Midwifery and Health Visiting (1998) *Midwives Rules and Code of Practice.* UKCC, London.

54 United Kingdom Central Council for Nursing, Midwifery and Health Visiting (1998) *Guidelines for Records and Record Keeping.* UKCC, London.

55 Maternal and Child Health Research Consortium (1997) *Confidential Enquiry into Stillbirths and Deaths in Infancy* (Fourth Annual Report). CESDI, London.

56 Maternal and Child Health Research Consortium (2001) *Confidential Enquiry into Stillbirths and Deaths in Infancy* (Eighth Annual Report). CESDI, London.

57 Bryne U (1999) Record keeping: a risk management perspective. *Br J Midwif.* **7** (7): 436–9.

58 Quilliam S (1999) Clinical risk management in midwifery: what are midwives for? *MIDIRS Midwif Digest.* **9** (3): 280–4.

59 Kirkham M (1999) The culture of midwifery in the National Health Service in England. *J Adv Nurs.* **30** (3): 732–9.

60 Kirkham M (2000) Midwives' support needs as childbirth changes. *J Adv Nurs.* **32** (2): 465–72.

Index